Surgical
Radiography

Surgical Radiography

Jamie E. Marlowe, R.T., B.A., M.B.A.
Technical Director
Department of Radiology
Fort Myers Community Hospital
Fort Myers, Florida

University Park Press • Baltimore

University Park Press
International Publishers in Medicine and Human Services
300 North Charles Street
Baltimore, Maryland 21201

Typeset by Ampersand, Inc.

Manufactured in the United States of America by Halliday Lithograph

Library of Congress Cataloging in Publication Data

Marlowe, Jamie E.
  Surgical radiography.

  Includes index.
  1. Surgery. 2. Diagnosis, Radioscopic. I. Title.
[DNLM: 1. Technology, Radiologic. 2. Radiography. WN 16C M349s]
RD31.5.M37 1983   617'.07572   83-6558
ISBN 0-8391-1831-7

*This book is affectionately dedicated to my Mother,
Grace Marlowe*

Contents

Preface

This book was written primarily for the student radiologic technologist; however, the experienced certified radiologic technologist may find that it can be used as a guide to certain procedures performed in the Operating Room.

This is not an exhaustive text. The exhaustive text often-times fails to satisfy many teachers and instructors of modern radiologic technology. There are many procedures in the surgical suite that are performed in the same manner as general radiographic procedures; however, these same procedures take on a drastic and profound change when performed within the realm and guidelines of an aseptic technique.

Frequently, the student radiologic technologist feels overwhelmed by the many formulas, techniques, and surgical restrictions imposed upon him; therefore, I have tried to explain and simplify these multiple restrictions so as to give the student a working edge prior to his or her arrival on the surgical scene.

In the main I have attempted to approach the technology and problems of surgical radiography in such a light as to demonstrate the importance as well as the gratification of the performance of good radiographic quality.

While it would be impossible to acknowledge all the help I have received in writing this book, I would like to especially thank:

Michael Kyle, M.D. who took the time to offer criticisms that resulted in many beneficial changes. It would be difficult to imagine this book going to publication without the help of Donald Gerson, M.D. His assistance was invaluable and the many interruptions he tolerated at the office and away from the office was far above the call of any academic duty. To Ms. Jean Tornello, R.N., for her immense help with the entire text. To the physicians on the surgical staff of Fort Myers Community Hospital for their many hours of discussion on surgical technique. I am extremely grateful to Lora West, R.T. who typed and retyped the manuscript. Without her this book would have been impossible. In addition, it is inconceivable that this text from beginning to end could have ever been accomplished without the sound advice, criticisms, and constructive recommendations of Ms. Dottie Fishburn. Indeed, she far exceeded any call of academic duty. I would certainly be remiss if I failed to acknowledge Lt. Anastasia Weber whose complete dedication for the completion of this text was unmatched. Her devotion to the radiological sciences has been exceeded only by her tremendous help during trying times. I will be eternally grateful for her many suggestions regarding this text and hold her solely responsible for the selection of the cover design.

I would also like to thank General Electric Medical Systems, North American Phillips (Medical Division), Eastman Kodak (Radiography Products), and E.I. Du Pont de Nemours (Radiographic Products Division), for their immense help and contributions.

All photographs are courtesy of Sam Johnson.

I sincerely hope that this book will be a contribution to the teaching of modern surgical radiography.

J.E.M.

Foreword

X-Rays have been used since the year of their discovery to search for and to document the extent of human disease. Many books are available for the technologist for routine radiological examination of non-surgical patients. The need has existed for a comprehensive textbook to include all aspects of surgical radiography. The author has achieved a well balanced presentation of the various facets of surgical radiography to present a uniform guideline to problem solving in various situations. An attempt has been made to achieve completeness without exhaustive and burdensome details.

The author, Jamie Marlowe, R.T., has drawn effectively and extensively upon his broad background of experience, and has to be congratulated for bringing together a well conceived, well executed concise textbook encompassing a difficult area in radiography.

Freddie P. Gargano, M.D.
Director of Radiology
Palmetto General Hospital
Hialeah, Florida and
Clinical Professor of Radiology
University of Miami School of Medicine
Miami, Florida

1

Asepsis

One of the many prerequisites to sound surgical radiography is a basic knowledge of aseptic technique. Although it is essential that the entire operating room suite be clean, whenever the skin or a mucous membrane is opened or a body cavity entered, all items contacting the patient or staff must be sterile. *Sterile means free of all living organisms*, especially the microorganisms responsible for infection. *The methods used to achieve and maintain a sterile field are collectively termed aseptic technique.* All items within a sterile field must be sterile. This is accomplished by subjecting the items to conditions that kill all organisms. The autoclave, which utilizes steam under pressure, and chemical sterilization with ethylene oxide gas are the most common methods used in hospitals (Figures 1-1 and 1-2).

Numerous methods of sterilization including radiation are used in commercial situations. Once an item is sterilized there must be an *antibacterial barrier* to prevent contamination. Various packaging materials are used for this purpose. Because any break in the integrity of the wrapping material would lead to contamination of the item, packages must be inspected carefully before opening for holes, tears, moisture, and expiration date. A contaminated package is not used within the sterile field.

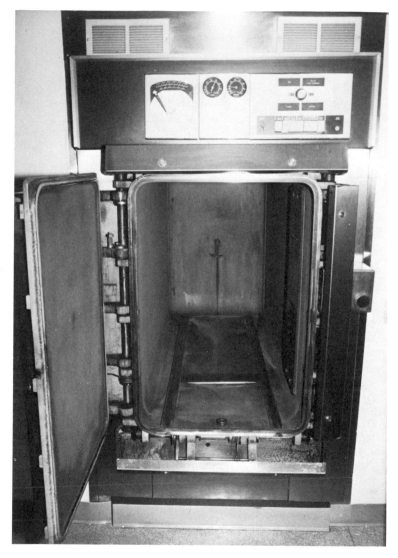

Figure 1-1. The autoclave: steam under pressure.

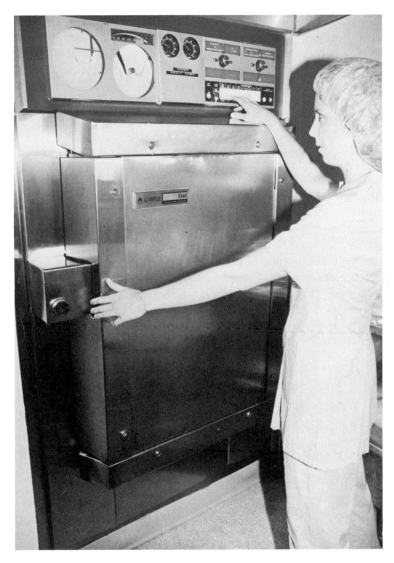

Figure 1-2. Sterilization with ethylene oxide gas.

The edges of the sterile containers are not considered sterile after they are opened. This applies as well to fluid-containing vessels; thus when solutions such as contrast media are poured, care must be taken not to allow solution to drip down the edges and then onto the sterile field.

Microorganisms are present on the skin surface of all humans and although *bacteria do not jump or fly*, they are carried on the dead skin cells that are constantly flaking off into the air. Operating room attire is designed to reduce the amount of air-borne contamination. The surgical team scrubs to reduce the number of organisms present on the hands and arms. Next, sterile gown and gloves are donned before the team members may enter the sterile field.

Sterile-attired persons and sterile items must contact only sterile areas. Likewise, persons without sterile attire and unsterile items must contact only unsterile areas. This means that the members of the surgical team, including the radiologic technologist, *must be aware of what is sterile and what is not sterile*, Surgical sterile gowns are worn by the surgeon, scrub nurse, and others on the sterile team. The areas considered sterile are the front from shoulder to table level and also the sleeves (Figures 1-3 and 1-4).

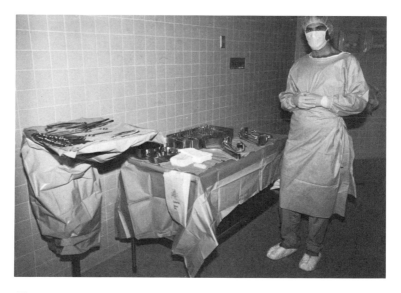

Figure 1-3. Gown considered sterile in front from shoulder to table level and also the sleeves.

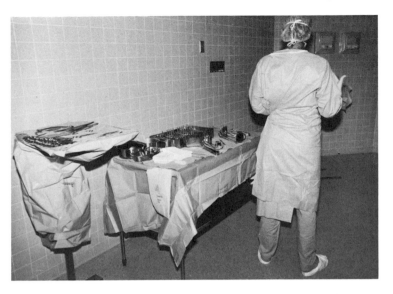

Figure 1–4. Sterile-attired scrub nurse. *Note*: The scrub gown worn by this nurse is considered sterile in the back as well as the front because of the type of gown. This type gown is known as a wrap-a-round.

The patient on the operating table is draped with sterile sheets to provide an antibacterial barrier between the patient and the sterile-attired team (Figure 1-5). Instrument tables are covered with sterile drapes. (Figures 1-6 and 1-7). These drapes are considered sterile only as far as the table level. Accessory items such as splash basins are draped to make them part of the sterile field (Figures 1-8 and 1-9).

All persons in the operating room without sterile attire must avoid all sterile-attired persons and sterile items by a safe margin. This safe margin is the distance required to avoid accidental contact and will vary with the size of the area.

Movement within and around the sterile field must not cause contamination. Sterile-attired persons should not enter into the traffic ways or leave the sterile area. Traffic should be limited, and only those persons who will participate in the operative procedure should be present in the operating room. When it is necessary for sterile-attired persons to pass each other, sterile should face sterile and unsterile face unsterile (Figure 1-10).

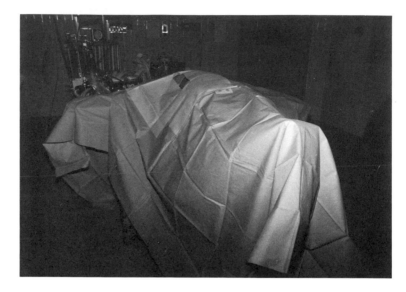

Figure 1-5. Patient on the operating table draped with sterile sheets.

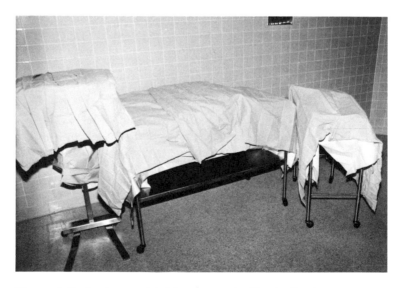

Figure 1-6. Instrument table covered with sterile drapes.

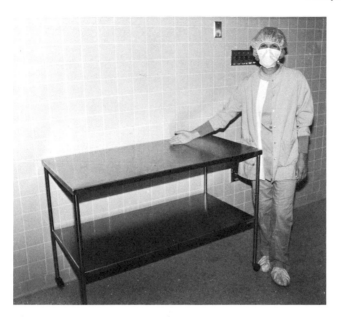

Figure 1-7. A bare instrument table.

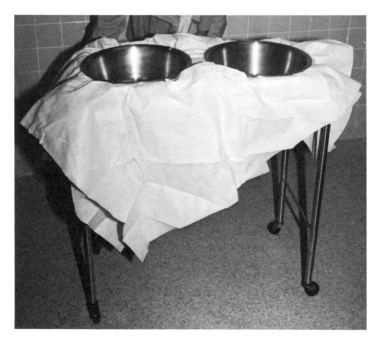

Figure 1-8. A sterile-draped stand with basins.

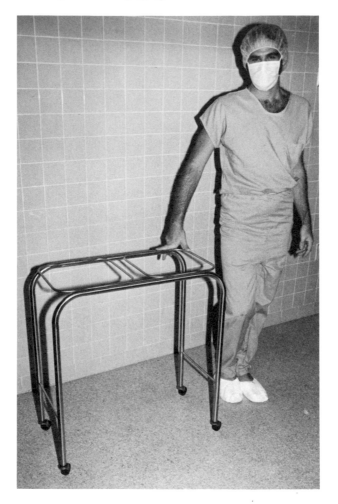

Figure 1-9. A bare stand without basin.

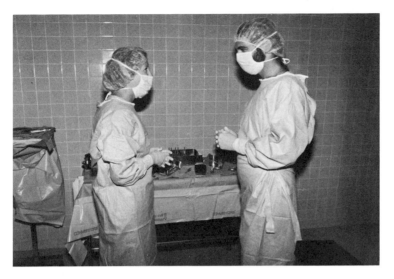

Figure 1-10. Sterile-attired persons pass face to face.

Persons without sterile attire should never reach across a sterile item or over the sterile field. Radiologic technologists must use care when placing cassettes or positioning the X-ray machine so that they do not violate the sterile field. When the radiologic technologist is unsure of the limits of the sterile field, he or she must always question the circulating nurse before proceeding. *When there is any doubt as to the sterility of an item*, it is considered contaminated and removed from the sterile field. Always report immediately any break in the sterile field such as contact with the sterile drapes or a splash basin.

Whenever antibacterial barriers are permeated by any moisture, contamination occurs. This is called *strike through*. Care must be taken to avoid contact of sterile items with solutions. Nonpermeable drapes are a protection against strike through.

Aseptic technique is an exercise in discipline. Remember, it is your responsibility to *learn* and *practice* aseptic technique.

ASEPTIC TECHNIQUE

The problem of dust and other microscopic debris falling from the X-ray tube into the sterile field is an inevitable consequence of two common mistakes. One is the failure to clean the X-ray machine properly with a cloth dampened by a surgically approved cleaning solution. The second is the failure to drape the X-ray machine with a sterile or at least a clean prefitting drape. Although there are commercially made drapes, such as Xomed, which is a transparent, packaged sterile drape, covering the X-ray tube, the use of a large Mayo cover suffices in most instances (Figures 1-11 and 1-12).

While C-Arm fluoroscopy is fairly well established in most operating theaters, it must be remembered that some hospitals continue to use the conventional portable X-ray machines, and unlike the C-Arm machine, they are not equipped with a sterile or autoclavable tube cover. Therefore, when using the conventional portable X-ray machine, the radiologic technologist should take the proper precautions to ensure good aseptic technique by cleaning and/or draping the machine to preclude any break in sterile technique.

Postsurgical cleaning of the X-ray apparatus is an important part of the continuing effort to ensure proper aseptic technique. If the X-ray machine is a permanent fixture, such as a ceiling-mounted unit in the operating room, then it should be thoroughly cleaned while not in use. If a portable X-ray machine is utilized for surgical procedures and is left in the operating suite after use, then it should be cleaned and draped so as to allow only the very minimum of dust and other nonsterile particles to contaminate not only the X-ray tube, but the entire machine. Usually a sheet or two sheets sewn together will amply cover the machine. It may well be that the hospital has its own laundry and linen facility, where a form-fitting cover for the X-ray machines can be sewed and outfitted.

Although covering these machines affords some protection against a break in aseptic technique, it does not mean that one can simply remove the cover and move the machine into the operating room and begin another surgical procedure. The machine should be cleaned again after removal of the cover prior to entering the operating room for the next X-ray exam.

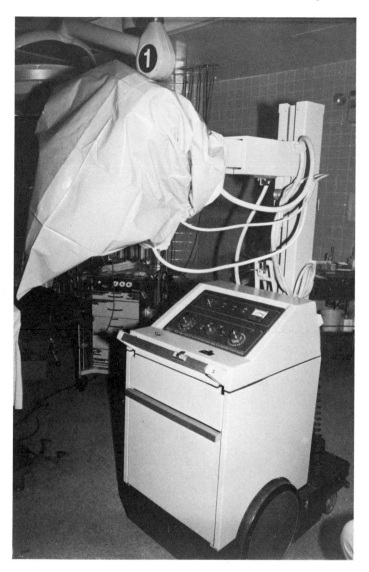

Figure 1-11. An X-ray tube housing draped with a sterile Mayo cover.

Notes

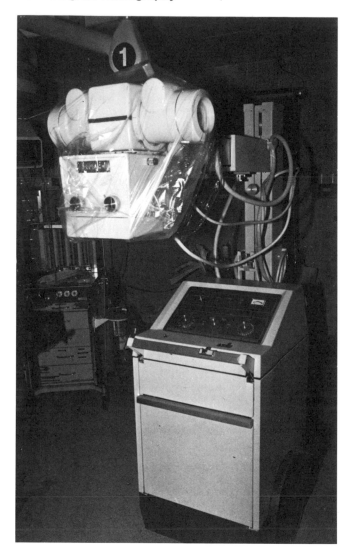

Figure 1-12. An X-ray tube housing with a sterile transparent drape.

There appears to be a great tendency for the operating room staff to call the surgical radiologic technologist at the last instant before the surgeon is ready for the X-ray exam and there seems to be little time for cleaning preparation. However, correct technique dictates that the machine be cleaned before entering the operating room and certainly before positioning the tube over the patient. Therefore, while covering the machine when not in use does not ensure total cleanliness, it does help in reducing time spent cleaning the machine prior to entering the operating room.

Maintaining cleanliness seems to be a never-ending process in the operating room and it does not end with cleaning only the X-ray machines. Cassettes, cassette holders, I.D. markers, and other X-ray accessories must be kept clean and in a usable condition. These accessories, particularly cassettes and cassette holders, must be thoroughly cleaned beause of their close proximity to the patient when a surgical radiographic examination is being performed. An unclean cassette, even though draped, in close proximity to a patient undergoing a hip operation can have drastic and devastating results on that patient's infection status.

SUMMARY

A dictum to sound surgical radiography is a basic knowledge of aseptic technique. Whenever the skin or a mucous membrane is opened or a body cavity entered, all items used must be sterile.

Sterile means free of all living organisms. The method used to achieve and maintain a sterile field is called aseptic technique. All items within a sterile field must be sterile. Steam under pressure and chemical sterilization with ethylene oxide gas are the most common methods used to sterilize items in a hospital.

Microorganisms are present on the skin of all humans, and although bacteria do not jump or fly, they are carried on the dead skin cells that are constantly flaking off into the air. Operating room attire is designed to reduce the amount of airborne contamination. The surgical team scrubs to reduce the number of organisms on the hands and arms. Sterile-attired persons and sterile items must contact only sterile areas.

Surgical gowns are considered sterile in the front from shoulder to table level and also the sleeves. The patient on the operating table is draped with sterile sheets to provide an antibacterial barrier. The distance required to avoid accidental contact with sterile items or sterile-attired persons is called the **safe margin**. Persons with unsterile attire should never reach across a sterile item or over the sterile field. When there is any doubt regarding the sterility of an item, it is considered contaminated.

Failure to drape and clean the X-ray machine properly results in a break of aseptic technique. Cassettes, cassette holders, I.D. markers, and other X-ray accessories must be kept clean and in a usable condition.

QUESTIONS

1. In relation to surgical asepsis, the term "sterile" means _____ .

2. The methods used to achieve and maintain a sterile field are called _____ .

3. The most common methods used in hospitals to sterilize surgical items are _____ .

4. Because microorganisms are present on the skin of all humans and although bacteria do not jump or fly, how are they present in the air?

5. What are the specific areas of the surgical gown that are considered sterile?

6. Why is the surgical patient on the operating table draped with sterile sheets?

7. All persons without sterile attire in the operating room must avoid all sterile attired persons and sterile items by a safe margin. What is the distance of this "safe margin"?

8. In what manner do sterile-attired persons pass each other?

9. Define "strike through."

10. The problem of dust and other microscopic debris falling from the X-ray tube into the sterile field is the result of two common mistakes. What are these two common mistakes?

2

Film Processing

Such a large volume of books, pamphlets, and scientific papers has been generated concerning film processing that one would think another published study on this subject superfluous. This is hardly true, because sound radiography begins and ends in the darkroom.

In this chapter the importance of the processing room (darkroom) in the surgical suite will be discussed. It must be remembered that, unlike the darkroom in the main radiology department, the darkroom in the surgical suite may not always be centrally located. It is obvious that the physical layout of the surgical suite varies from hospital to hospital, and hence so does the location of the X-ray darkroom. The centrally located surgical X-ray darkroom will yield greater efficiency.

Usually the X-ray darkroom in surgery is a small unit situated in an obscure corner of the operating suite. This can be a great disadvantage in terms of time, as we shall see in a later chapter. The handicaps resulting from a poorly placed darkroom are numerous. It is time consuming for the radiologic technologist to walk to and from the operating room. It is tiring to transport cassettes from one end of the surgical suite to the other. Most of all, it is unfair to the patient under general anesthesia. The student technologist must be constantly aware of the patient under general anesthesia and utilize his or her time to the patient's advantage. Thus the placement of the surgical darkroom does play a large part in the patient's welfare.

There are many factors other than location to consider when planning the surgical darkroom-such as adequate ventilation, construction of light-tight doors, readily accessible electrical and plumbing conduits, pass boxes, safe lights, and storage facilities, to name a few.

The surgical darkroom must be large enough to accommodate developer and fixer replenishment tanks. Ideally a backup system of wet tanks should be present and prepared for emergency use in the event of a power failure or other unforeseen breakdowns of automatic processing.

Automatic or rapid processing has become an important aspect of modern surgical radiography. One can select from among several different models of rapid processing equipment. The model best suited for a given operating room will depend on many factors related to that particular operating room, including the number of radiologic surgically related cases performed daily and the specific types of surgical procedures performed, insofar as this relates to the use of a particular film size. As more radiographic processing chemicals are used to develop or process larger size X-ray film (such as 14 × 17 or 11 × 14), it is important to install the rapid processing machine that will accommodate film of that size. (Figure 2-1).

Mixing valves to maintain correct water temperature are essential for a rapid processing machine that will handle a large volume of films on a daily basis. The radiologic technologist must be familiar with this equipment in order to make minor adjustments in any given situation (Figure 2-2).

The reliability of the automatic processor in the surgical suite is of paramount importance. Therefore, care must be taken to ensure a desirable preventive maintenance program. Water filters must be replaced at correct intervals. Transport rollers must be cleaned on a daily basis and inspected for wear on the roller gears. Chemical levels must be inspected daily and replenished as needed. A proper preventive maintenance program is not only desirable, it is essential, as it will spare many hours of nonprocessing time and hence avoid the ill feelings of the surgical staff.

In conclusion, it must be remembered that the breakdown of a processor being used for surgical radiography does not

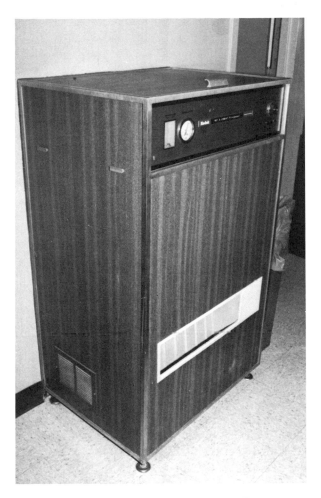

Figure 2-1. A Kodak automatic rapid film processor.

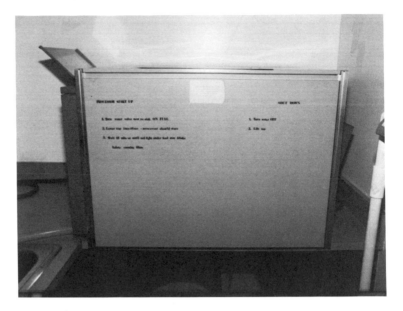

Figure 2-2. A small automatic processor such as the one shown above is sufficient for a light to moderately busy surgery department.

simply involve repairing the processor and repeating an anterior-posterior view of the skull or a lateral chest film. It involves, in addition, a complicated explanation to the surgeon why he or she must reinject a gall bladder that has already been removed and sent to the laboratory for a frozen section report. Unlike film processing in the main radiology department, there may only be one opportunity in the surgical suite. Therefore, film processing must be considered one of the most important aspects of sound surgical radiography.

SUMMARY

The location of the processing room in the surgical suite is important, because of the time required to transport X-ray film from the operating room to the darkroom for development. It has been shown that time-saving steps are important to help minimize the actual time the patient is under anesthesia.

QUESTIONS

1. The processing room in the surgical suite should be
_____ located.

2. List the handicaps encountered in having a poorly located processing room in the surgical suite.

3. List six considerations to think of when dealing with the surgical darkroom other than location.
   1.
   2.
   3.
   4.
   5.
   6.

4. In the event of a power failure or other unforseen processor breakdown, what processing system must be readily available?

3

The Portable X-ray Machine in Surgery

With the advent of Roentgen's X-rays came the inevitable birth of surgical radiology and, consequently, surgical radiography.

In modern surgical radiography, in larger institutions the use of the single-unit portable X-ray machine is quickly diminishing and has been superceded by other methods and X-ray equipment. However, in smaller hospitals the single unit not only thrives, but is an integral part of surgical radiography. While the larger hospitals utilize sophisticated and expensive equipment (discussed at length in Chapter 5), such as C-arm fluoroscopy and overhead-mounted ceiling tubes for their surgical radiologic needs, it must be remembered that the smaller institutions cannot financially afford to purchase such equipment. Therefore, the single-unit portable continues to be utilized, and in most instances with very reliable and desirable results.

The basis for the use of the single-unit portable X-ray apparatus in surgical radiography is the fact that with the exception of C-arm fluoroscopy, the single-unit portable X-ray machine will usually produce the same radiographic results as ceiling or other mounted X-ray apparatus with comparable milliamperage and kilovoltage potentials. This is to say that a

Notes

200 MaS, 150 KvP portable X-ray machine will produce the same results as a 200 MaS, 150 KvP ceiling-mounted X-ray machine. All other factors, such as screen speed, distance, developing and fixing chemical temperature, patient size, etc., must be constant. In most instances a portable X-ray machine of lower milliamperage and kilovoltage potential will produce the same results, for practical purposes, as a permanent or ceiling-mounted X-ray apparatus of high milliamperage and kilovoltage. There is no doubt that radiographic quality is greater with higher milliamperage and kilovoltage than with lower values; however, the end result, that is, the diagnostic yield of the radiograph, is such that the radiologist or surgeon can derive sufficient diagnostic information from the study to interpret correctly the radiographic examination.

In essence, correct utilization of distance, chemical temperature, processing time, screen and film speed will generally yield a radiograph as diagnostically productive from a portable X-ray unit of less MaS–KvP potential as it will from a mounted X-ray machine with greater MaS–KvP potential.

A portable X-ray machine with a 300 MaS–125 KvP output will suffice in most cases involving surgical radiologic examinations. This type of portable X-ray unit has sufficient radiation output to penetrate even the most obese patients. While it is bulky and cumbersome, and often time consuming to use, it does produce fine quality radiographs, and the diagnostic information derived more than outweighs the inconvenience caused by the size of a machine with this amount of radiation output. Usually two portable X-ray machines of this type are kept in the surgical suite for use during hip nailing radiography and as a backup unit. In addition, surgical cases that are being performed simultaneously require the use of these machines. Therefore, it is almost essential that two machines be available at all times. Machines of this size are operated from a 220-volt outlet and will not function from a 110-volt outlet (Figures 3-1 and 3-2).

Portable X-ray machines that are smaller in size and radiation output will function from either a 110-volt outlet, or a 220-volt outlet, and will produce radiographs of fine radiographic and diagnostic value. These smaller machines are easy to move about and tube positioning is fairly easy.

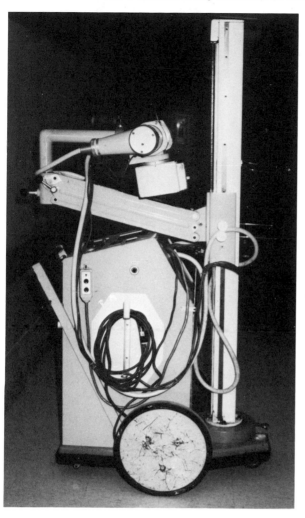

Figure 3-1. Portable X-ray machine utilizing a 110-volt outlet.

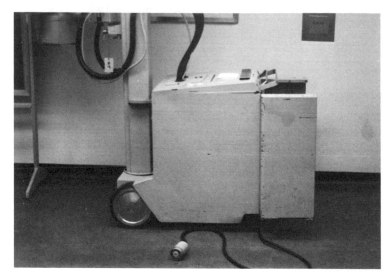

Figure 3-2. A portable X-ray machine that will operate only on a 220-volt outlet.

Not only are they ideal for surgical cases, such as open and closed reductions of fractured extremities, but they are often preferred by the radiologic technologist. Generally they are preferred because of their maneuverability, but many radiologic technologists favor their use because of the small size and the ease with which they can be positioned in the smaller operating room.

Although manufacturers of X-ray machines have made great strides in producing better, lighter, smaller, and more maneuverable equipment, there is a constant effort to produce and supply the ultimate portable X-ray machine. In this chapter we will discuss many of the advantages, as well as disadvantages, of the battery-energized unit and the capacitor discharge unit (Figures 3-3 and 3-4).

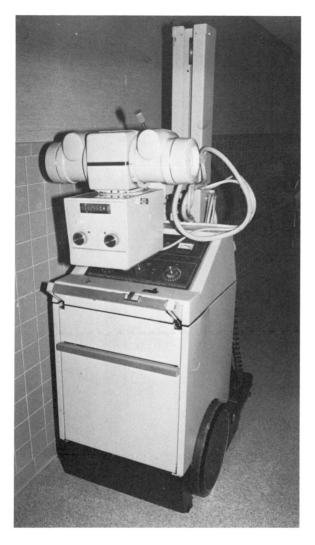

Figure 3-3. A battery-energized portable X-ray unit.

Notes

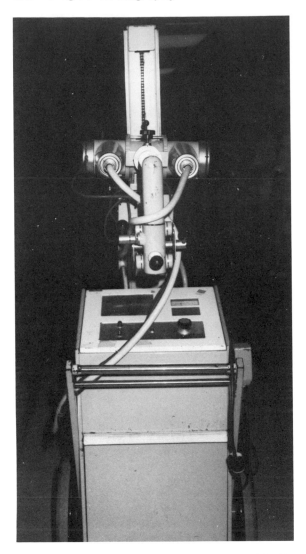

Figure 3-4. A capacitor discharge portable X-ray unit.

The capacitor discharge unit and the battery-energized unit operate on the principle of stored energy. Let us start with the capacitor discharge unit which stores a quantity of electricity in a capacitor (condenser) and then discharges this stored energy through an X-ray tube. When using the capacitor discharge unit, the kilovoltage value decreases during an exposure. Therefore, the penetrating power of the X-rays decreases.

The capacitor discharge unit is usually designed to control the maximum kilovoltage drop so that it does not exceed 30%. Therefore, to avoid unnecessary skin dosage to the patient, the exposure is started at 100 Kv and is terminated at about 70 Kv.

The main advantage of the capacitor discharge unit over the conventional portable two-pulse unit is its lower current demand. Conventional portable or mobile X-ray units require an electrical outlet that will permit the use of high currents and this may not always be readily available in the operating room. The capacitor discharge unit bypasses this problem by the utilization of a high-capacity condenser and can be charged and ready for an exposure in a matter of seconds.

During the exposure the stored energy in the capacitor discharge unit is discharged within a few hundredths or tenths of a second, making the unit extremely attractive for surgical radiographic studies. A 300 MA capacitor discharge unit compares favorably in performance with a 500 MA two-pulse unit. Many of the units are self-propelled, powered by a lead-acid battery-operated motor. The capacitor discharge unit is easily maneuvered and usually of moderate size.

The battery-energized unit, like the capacitor discharge unit is used for the production of X-rays without the necessity of a special electrical receptacle. The battery-energized unit, like the capacitor discharge unit, is self-propelled, powered by a lead-acid or other type battery-operated motor. Compared with the capacitor discharge unit, the battery-energized unit has a greater energy storage capacity. The battery-energized unit has enough energy for a series of exposures, whereas the capacitor discharge unit must be charged after each exposure.

The greatest disadvantage of the battery-energized unit is the necessity of recharging the batteries after a series of exposures This is a definite disadvantage in the operating room, as a patient in need of immediate surgery cannot wait for the charging of batteries.

The battery-energized unit produces a higher MaS value than the capacitor discharge unit; this is because the capacitor discharge unit is limited by the condenser.

The one great advantage of the battery-energized unit, as opposed to the capacitor discharge unit or conventional portable X-ray machine, is the ability to use the battery-energized unit without an electrical receptacle. The need for an external power supply is completely eliminated (except to recharge the batteries) by the use of storage batteries. This feature becomes extremely attractive during a power failure. While it is true that most hospitals are equipped with emergency generators that are immediately energized during a power failure, the energy drain is such that the number of electrical receptacles and amount of energy being used is significant. Therefore, the readily available portable X-ray machine that does not require an external power supply definitely has a place in the operating room.

In comparing the capacitor discharge unit with the battery-energized unit, the different energy sources dictate the varying performance characteristics. Some of the technical aspects and comparisons are listed below.

	Battery-energized unit	Capacitor discharge unit
External power supply required	No	Yes
Maximum output per exposure at 100 Kv	300 MaS	30 MaS
Delay between series exposures	Several hours	Negligible
Delay between single exposures	Negligible	5–10 seconds
Weight of the X-ray unit	High to very high	High
Exposure time at equal MaS load	Long	Short
X-ray tube current	100 MA	200–400 MA

It is evident that both the capacitor discharge unit and the battery-energized unit have a place in the operating room and in radiology in general.

It is hoped that the student will learn the different mechanisms of the two units discussed above and will utilize them to their best advantage in different situations. Once again, it is imperative that the technologist use the particular technique and equipment that are the most advantageous for the patient in any given situation.

SUMMARY

In modern surgical radiography, the use of the single-unit portable X-ray machine is quickly diminishing and has been superceded by other methods and X-ray equipment in larger institutions. However, in smaller hospitals the single unit not only thrives, but is an integral part of surgical radiography. Therefore, the single-unit portable X-ray machine continues to be utilized and, in most instances, with very reliable and desirable results.

The basis of the use of the single-unit portable X-ray apparatus in surgical radiography is the fact that with the exception of C-arm fluoroscopy, the single-unit portable X-ray machine will usually produce the same radiographic results as ceiling or other mounted X-ray apparatus with the comparable milliamperage and kilovoltage potentials.

Correct utilization of distance, chemistry, temperature, processing time, screen and film speed will yield a radiograph as diagnostically productive from a portable X-ray unit of less MaS–KvP potential as it will from a mounted X-ray machine with greater MaS–KvP potential.

It is also important that two portable X-ray machines be kept in the surgical suite for use during a hip nailing or as a backup unit in situations such as simultaneous surgical procedures.

The capacitor discharge unit and the battery-energized unit operate on the principle of stored energy. A quantity of electricity is stored in a capacitor (condenser) which then is discharged through the X-ray tube. In the case of the capacitor discharge unit the kilovoltage value decreases during an exposure. Therefore, the penetrating power of the X-rays decreases. The main advantage of the capacitor discharge unit

Notes

over the conventional portable two-pulse unit is its lower current demand. When an exposure is made with the capacitor discharge unit, the stored energy is discharged in a few hundredths or tenths of a second.

The battery-energized unit, like the capacitor discharge unit, is used for the production of X-rays without the necessity of a special electrical receptacle. The battery-energized unit has enough energy for a series of exposures, whereas the capacitor discharge unit must be charged after each exposure. The greatest disadvantage of the battery-energized unit is the necessity of recharging the batteries after a series of exposures. The battery-energized unit produces a higher MaS value than the capacitor discharge unit; this is because the capacitor discharge unit is limited by the condenser.

In comparing the capacitor discharge unit with the battery-energized unit, the different energy sources dictate the varying performance characteristics.

QUESTIONS

1. The capacitor discharge unit and the battery energized unit operate on what principle?

2. When using the capacitor discharge unit, the kilovoltage value decreases during an exposure. How does this effect the penetrating power of the X-rays?

3. The capacitor discharge unit is usually manufactured to control the maximum kilovoltage drop so as not to exceed what percentage?

4. What is the main advantage of the capacitor discharge unit over the conventional portable two-pulse unit?

5. Why is the capacitor discharge unit extremely attractive for surgical radiographic studies?

6. A 300 MA capacitor discharge unit compares favorably in performance with a
   a. 200 MA–two-pulse unit
   b. 300 MA–two-pulse unit
   c. 500 MA–two-pulse unit

7. During the exposure, the stored energy in the capacitor discharge unit is discharged in a few
   a. hundredths or tenths of a second
   b. seconds
   c. minutes

8. Which has a greater energy storage capacity?
   a. battery-energized unit
   b. capacitor discharge unit

9. What is the greatest disadvantage of the battery-energized unit?

10. Why does the battery-energized unit produce a higher MaS value than the capacitor discharge unit?

11. What is the one great advantage of the battery energized unit, as opposed to the capacitor discharge unit or conventional portable X-ray machine?

12. What is the maximum output per exposure at 100 Kv of the battery-energized unit? The capacitor discharge unit?

13. What is the delay between series exposures of the battery-energized unit? The capacitor discharge unit?

14. What is the delay between single exposures of the battery-energized unit? The capacitor discharge unit?

4

Postoperative Foreign Bodies

A foreign body in a patient is defined as any object within the body that is not a natural part of or that has not grown in the body (such as a neoplasm). In other words, any inanimate object that is in the chest or abdominal cavity or that has passed through the skin and is embedded in the tissue is considered a foreign body.

In this chapter a certain type of foreign body will be discussed: a surgical sponge or instrument left in the patient's chest or abdominal cavity following surgery.

It has been, and is still, the practice of surgeons and surgical teams to count all surgical sponges prior to any operation. Before the first scalpel blade even touches the surgical patient, each sponge, regardless of size or configuration, is counted simultaneously by two people, and duly recorded on the patient's operative chart or sheet. This practice is not limited to surgical sponges, however. It includes the systematic counting of surgical clamps, hemostats, scissors, and, in short, all surgical instruments involved or utilized in that particular surgical procedure or operation. The sponges and instruments are counted again at the end of the procedure and must tally with the initial count. This is a tedious and time-consuming

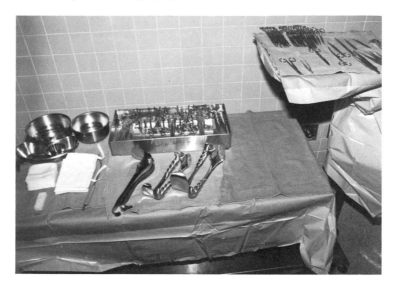

Figure 4–1. A major surgical setup.

effort, but one that must be observed in order to ensure patient safety. A major surgical "set-up" is shown in Figure 4-1. Despite these precautions, mistakes do occur. Thus a postoperative abdominal X-ray is usually taken in the operating suite just before closing the incision when a patient has undergone an abdominal operation to check for sponges or instruments that may have been inadvertently left in the abdomen.

When surgery of other parts of the body is performed a postoperative X-ray of that particular part of the anatomy is taken to demonstrate the postoperative status. This postoperative radiologic examination is popularly referred to as a "closing film," and is becoming increasingly popular as a means of preventing foreign bodies from being left in patients.

Modern medicine offers a fairly large number and variety of surgical sponges. The appearance of these sponges is completely different in a dry state than in a wet state (Figures 4-2 and 4-3).

These sponges not only demonstrate a profound difference in physical appearance from the dry state to the wet state, as previously mentioned, but are decidedly different in appear-

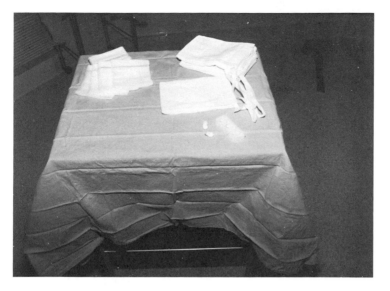

Figure 4-2. Most surgical sponges presented in dry state.

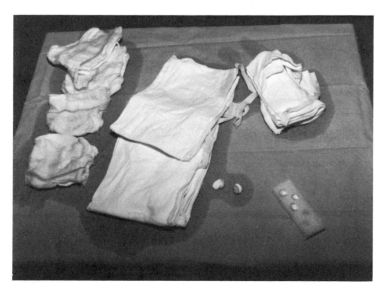

Figure 4-3. Most major surgical sponges presented in a wet state.

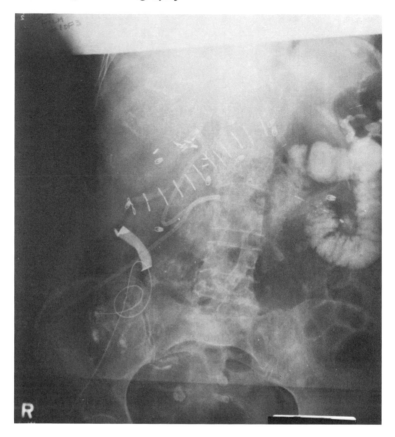

Figure 4-4. An X-ray film demonstrating a surgical sponge inadvertently left in the patient's body.

ance and configuration when outside the body as opposed to in situ (Figure 4-4).

A comparative study of the radiologic appearance of the sponges used in a given hospital may be helpful to the radiologist and surgeon. The study can be carried out by utilizing the following method. Place each sponge on a clear X-ray film in its dry state and secure it by transparent tape. This will be the "dry state control exhibit." Next, using a completely new set of sponges, wet each sponge and squeeze the sponges and place them on a 14 × 17 cassette for table top technique radiography. After taking X-ray films of the sponges, label the completed X-ray and retain this X-ray for comparative use. These comparative study films are often helpful in identifying the sponge on postoperative radiographic examinations (Figure 4-5).

The radiologic technologist and student radiologic technologist must be observant when performing postoperative studies. Most of the studies are performed while the patient is on the operating table, just prior to closure of the surgical wound, and sponges can be inadvertently left upon the patient

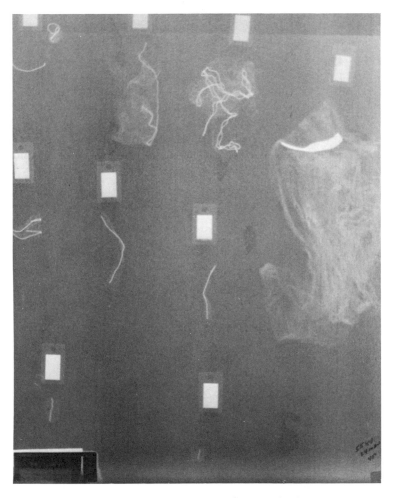

Figure 4-5. An X-ray film of most major surgical sponges.

and obscured by a surgical drape. In that case, they will not really be inside the patient, although it will appear so on the film. The radiologic technologist must be observant when performing the postoperative closing film, to prevent this confusing situation.

SUMMARY

Any inanimate object that is in the chest or abdominal cavity or that has passed through the integumentary system and is embedded in the tissue is considered a foreign body.

It is the practice of surgeons and surgical teams to count all surgical sponges prior to any operation and at the termination of the procedure, to prevent their being left in the patient.

The postoperative radiologic examination referred to as the "closing film" provides an additional safeguard against this and is becoming increasingly popular.

Modern surgery utilizes a fairly large number and variety of surgical sponges and these sponges are detectable and identifiable by radiologic examination.

QUESTIONS

1. Define foreign body.

2. Describe how surgical sponges are detected on X-rays.

3. An X-ray generally taken just before surgical closure following an operation is referred to as _____.

4. What should the radiologic technologist be careful of when taking this postoperative X-ray?

5. What routine do the operating room teams follow before and after each and every operation involving chest or abdominal surgery?

6. Every radiology department should have on hand a guide to inform the radiologist exactly what type sponges are used in surgery. Explain how this guide is obtained.

7. The guide to sponges used in surgical procedures should include _____ and _____ states.

5

Surgical C-arm Fluoroscopy

Surgical C-arm fluoroscopy has been in use for the past 20 years. Since its inception many innovations and improvements have been developed, but the basic concept, that of an X-ray tube and fluoroscopic image intensifier mounted on opposite ends of a C-shaped movable gantry, remains the same. This arrangement allows fluoroscopy of a patient lying on a pedestal table at multiple positions and angles without touching or moving the patient. The C-arm fluoroscopic unit is regarded as an essential piece of equipment in modern radiology and is widely used throughout the United States and Europe. Two types of units exist; portable and ceiling-mounted. While the portable unit finds use today in fluoroscopy for pacemaker implantation in the intensive care ward and for peripheral lung biopsy, C-arm fluoroscopy still has its widest use in the operating room, where the ceiling-mounted or portable unit is used for surgical fluoroscopy, the purpose for which it was originally invented (Figure 5-1).

Fiber optics play an important role in the image quality of some of the newer C-arm fluoroscopic units, and the single most important advantage of these is superior image quality. Before the use of fiber optics, surgeons were forced to work with inferior fluoroscopic images, and often this resulted in erroneous radiographic interpretations. Image quality depends on quantum noise and resolution; high absorption, improved

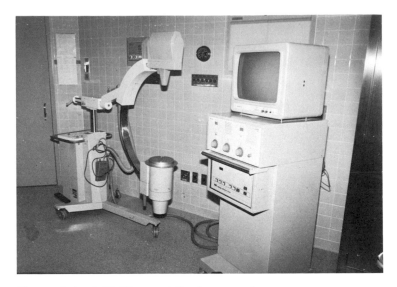

Figure 5-1. A Phillips mobile C-arm unit.

electron optics, and better screen design, paired with fiber optic coupling, have decreased quantum noise and improved resolution—leading to better image quality in modern C-arm units.

The radiation output of any fluoroscopic unit is always of great concern, and this is certainly true of a unit being used by nonradiologists. The surgical radiologic technologist, in this case, must be particularly concerned with radiation exposure to him or herself, since he/she must often be present during fluoroscopic examinations.

The radiation output of the mobile C-arm fluoroscopic unit varies from 20 MA at 90 KvP to 100 MA at 100 KvP. These values are more than adequate to penetrate the average and above-average size patient. The ceiling-mounted C-arm fluoroscopic unit can accommodate even the largest patients. Ceiling-mounted units have few limitations with regard to MaS and KvP. These can be equipped with heavy-duty tubes and transformers and a rotating anode, just as in any other radiographic or fluoroscopic X-ray room, and the radiation output is then in the 100–1000 MA range. It must be noted that most of the mobile C-arm fluoroscopic units are equipped with stationary anodes. Again, there is considerable variation

between the above-mentioned units in terms of anodes, MaS, **Notes**
and KvP, and it is difficult to establish generalizations regarding these MaS–KvP values. Mobile and ceiling mounted
C-arm fluoroscopic units exhibit similar general traits fluoroscopically, but radiographically, they can be, and often are,
quite dissimilar. We will learn more about the ceiling-mounted
C-arm fluoroscopy unit and portable units later in this
chapter.

Thus far, we have spoken of the C-arm fluoroscopic unit
only in terms of its KvP, MaS, radiation output, and anodes;
now let us turn our attention to equipment design and
equipment geometry. While most experienced radiologic
technologists tend to speak of the motion of the C-arm unit in
terms of arc movement, free space in arc, arc depth, wig-wag,
horizontal travel, etc., these terms are not easily understood by
the student who has recently begun his radiologic education;
therefore, more common terms will be used in the description
that follows.

The C-arm fluoroscopic unit is capable of many different
types of positioning, by virtue of its design. The angulation of
the X-ray beam can be altered by sliding the C-arm through
the sleeve (Figure 5-2). Through height adjustment, the C-arm

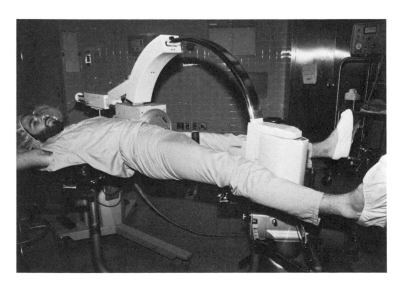

Figure 5-2. An altered X-ray beam caused by sliding the tube
head through the sleeve.

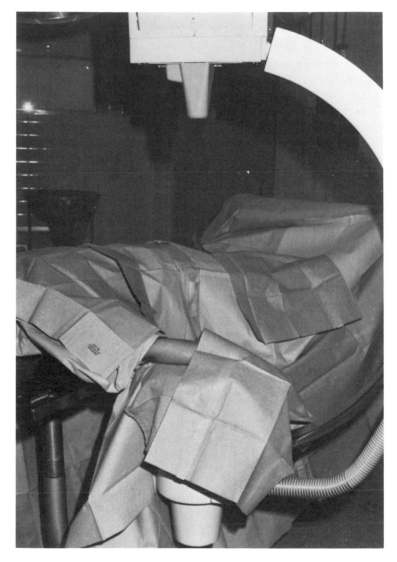

Figure 5-3A. Vertical movement of the C-arm (draped to indicate sterile field).

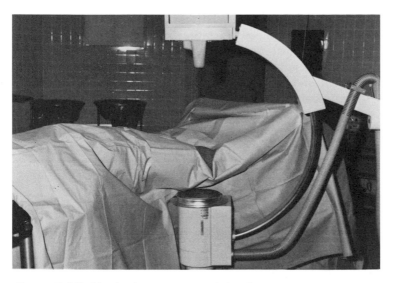

Figure 5-3B. Vertical movement of the C-arm.

can be moved horizontally toward or away from the patient (Figures 5-3A and B). Horizontal, vertical, and swiveling movements enable scanning of large areas without moving the stand. The short construction of the image intensifier–T.V. camera combination greatly reduces the possibility of collision with the operating lamp or, in the undertable technique, with the operating table. These features become important when actual surgical procedures are being performed and the radiologic technologist is actively involved in the radiologic aspects of the case. The use of the C-arm unit in specific types of surgery will be covered in greater detail in ensuing chapters on operative urology, surgery of the extremities, operative cholangiography, hip nailing radiography, and fluoroscopy.

We will now turn to a comparison of the ceiling-mounted and portable C-arm fluoroscopic units. In contrast to the mobile C-arm fluoroscopic unit, the ceiling-mounted unit has few limitations in terms of radiation output. This is because larger X-ray generators can be utilized with a unit that is not self-contained. The maneuverability of the C-arm of the ceiling-mounted unit, whether it is fluoroscopic or diagnostic, is in most cases greater than that of the mobile unit. The space occupied by the two units differs. The ceiling-mounted unit occupies no space below the table level, of course, whereas the mobile unit necessarily occupies floor space at a premium in the operating suite, which is usually already overcrowded with equipment and personnel.

Video recorders can be coupled to the C-arm unit and have been in use for a fairly long period of time in radiology. While several different commercial models are available, offering various imaging options, the details of their mode of operation hold little interest for the student technologist. Therefore, only the general mechanism and features of these devices will be described here.

Essentially, the video recorder is capable of magnetically storing fluoroscopic television images, usually on a rotating metallic disc. These images can then be "called back" and displayed for any length of time on the T.V. monitor, either as single, "still" images, or in some models as short sequences of "live-action" fluoroscopy (the sequence usually can be played back in variable slow motion or in "stop-action" motion). In short, the video recorder offers a form of "instant replay" (Figure 5-4).

The chief advantage of this is in the reduction of radiation exposure to the patient and personnel operating the fluoroscopic unit. For example, if a surgeon wishes to study a given fluoroscopic image for 30 seconds, he does not need to keep his foot on the fluoroscopy pedal, and thus expose the patient for 30 seconds. Instead, he can store the desired fluoroscopic image on the video recorder, play back the image on the T.V. monitor, and study it for as long as he wishes without further exposing the patient. This technique of short-exposure fluoroscopy with concurrent video recording of single "still" images is referred to as "electronic radiography," and can reduce radiation dose by as much as 95% over conventional fluoroscopy.

In spite of the technical complexities of the C-arm fluoroscopic unit and the disc recorders that couple with the unit, it is relatively easy to master their operation. It is the responsibility of the radiologic technologist to learn and master the use of such units to ensure patient safety, speed in performing operative radiologic studies, and production of diagnostic radiographs for the radiologist and surgeon.

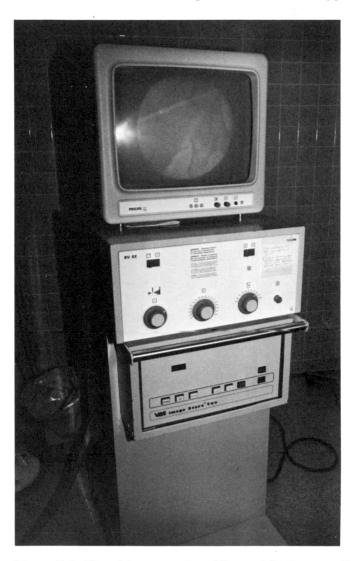

Figure 5-4. The video recorder of the mobile C-arm unit.

In conclusion, the radiologic technologist and the student radiologic technologist must be constantly aware of the fact that there is no substitute for anything less than optimal radiographs, particularly in terms of the welfare of the patient under anesthetic agents.

The mobile C-arm fluoroscopic unit and the C-arm fluroscopic and diagnostic ceiling-mounted unit are precision machines that can help produce positive results in all of the above situations when properly utilized.

SUMMARY

Surgical C-arm fluoroscopy has been in use for the past 20 years. The C-arm fluoroscopic unit has a specially designed configuration, much like the letter "C", hence the name. Two basic types of C-arm fluoroscopic units are in use today. One is a portable, or mobile unit, the other a ceiling-mounted unit. Both units are image intensifiers fluoroscopically. Fiber optics play an important role in the image quality of the C-arm fluoroscopic unit.

The radiation output of the mobile C-arm fluoroscopic unit varies from 20 MA at 90 KvP to 100 Ma at 100 KvP. The ceiling-mounted units have few limitations in MaS and KvP, as a result of the separate X-ray generators that can accommodate these ceiling-mounted units.

The C-arm fluoroscopic unit affords many different types of fluoroscopic positioning, by virtue of its design, and this flexibility becomes important when actual surgical cases are being performed.

There are video recorders that can be coupled to the C-arm fluoroscopic units, allowing great reductions in radiation exposure to the patient and operating room personnel.

QUESTIONS

1. For what use was the C-arm fluoroscopic unit designed?

2. Name two radiologic studies for which the mobile C-arm fluoroscopic unit is used in the intensive care ward.

3. Name two factors on which the C-arm fluoroscopic unit image quality is dependent.

4. Briefly explain the term "electronic radiography."

6

Operative Cholangiography

Surgical or operative cholangiography was first performed by Mirizzi in 1930.

    On the basis of the author's observations and the reports of other workers, one arrives at the definite conclusion that it has gained wide attention and varying degrees of popularity. Operative cholangiography is based on a combination of surgical and radiologic procedures that permit visualization of the biliary tract.

    Some surgeons perform operative cholangiography as a matter of routine, whereas others are rather selective in utilizing the procedure. Whatever the case may be, the radiologic technologist plays a critical role in the operative cholangiography procedure.

    To obtain optimum radiographs when performing an operative cholangiogram, the radiologic technologist must understand biliary tract anatomy. The bile ducts are divided into three major portions: the cystic, the common hepatic, and the common bile including its terminal portion at the ampulla of Vater. The minor portions include the right and left hepatic ducts with their corresponding radicles (Figure 6-1).

    The biliary tract is visualized during operative cholangiography by injection of contrast material through a catheter placed in the cystic duct. The gall bladder is removed and a small diameter catheter is introduced into the remnant of the

Notes

53

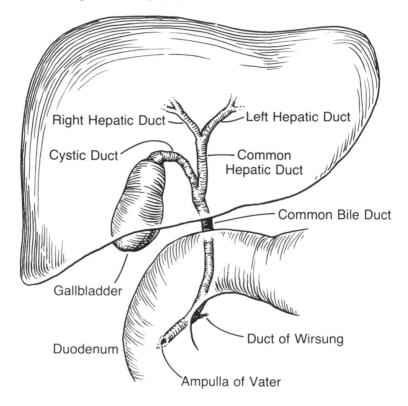

Figure 6-1. The biliary tree.

cystic duct; a suture is then placed and tied so as to prevent the catheter from losing its position.

As has been mentioned several times throughout this text, time is an important factor in any surgical procedure, and this is true during operative cholangiography. Because of the time factor, that is, keeping the patient anesthetized no longer than necessary, certain techniques should be employed prior to anesthetizing the patient. The patient should be positioned prior to the introduction of anesthesia, with the left side elevated 15 to 20 degrees. Because operative cholangiography is performed with the patient in the supine position, the elevation of the patient in the above-described manner will place the patient in the right posterior oblique (RPO) position.

This position will in most cases prevent superimposition of the spine and the region of the bile ducts.

With the manufacture of better and superior grids, the Bucky Tray in the operating room has become obsolete. The one exception is the cysto table, which will be discussed in a following chapter. Therefore, a cassette tunnel is used in most cases. The cassette tunnel may be a portable unit or it may be built into the more modern operating tables.

After this portion of the surgical procedure or operation is completed the operative cholangiogram is then performed in the following manner.

Place the grid cassette in a cassette holder that fits and will slide into and through a tunnel trough. Position the cassette so that the base of the cassette is six inches above the iliac crest; then position the cassette so that the lateral edge coincides with the lateral aspect of the patient's body.

CENTRAL RAY

Direct the central ray perpendicularly to the midpoint of the cassette. It must be remembered that the gall bladder itself is not the main structure to be visualized when performing operative cholangiography. In fact, more often that not, the gall bladder has been removed. The structures being demonstrated are the various biliary ducts and their radicles. Therefore, a greater area must be demonstrated when performing operative cholangiography than is required in a simple oral cholecystogram.

Another important factor to remember when performing operative cholangiography is the suspension of the patient's respiration. Apnea is induced by the anesthesiologist or anesthetist and is not controlled by the surgical radiologic technologist. Therefore, some communication must take place between the anesthesiologist and radiologic technologist, anesthesiologist and surgeon, or anesthetist and surgeon prior to radiographic exposure. Someone must be responsible for giving the command when the patient's respiration has been suspended. If this is not done, then the entire radiologic examination becomes folly, as the structures to be demonstrated are obscured by respiratory motion, resulting in a

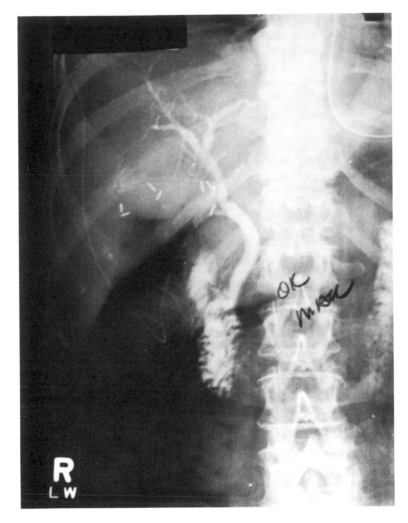

Figure 6-2. Operative cholangiogram without T-tube.

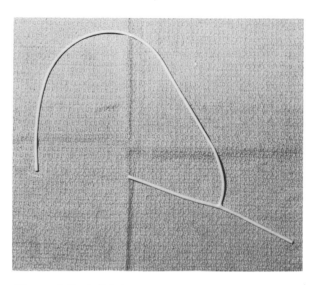

Figure 6-3. A T-tube.

worthless radiographic examination. The anesthesiologist usually signals the surgeon that apnea has been induced and in turn the surgeon directs the surgical radiologic technologist to make the radiographic exposure.

It is not enough to assume that the surgeon or the anesthesiologist will give the command to make the radiographic exposure. The surgical radiologic technologist must speak with either the anesthesiologist or the surgeon and definitely know which person will be giving directions. Remember, the patient is under the influence of anesthetic agents and, as stressed so often in this text, time is of the essence.

After the film has been developed, it should be immediately returned to the operating room for initial viewing by the surgeon (Figure 6-2). The surgeon may require additional filming based on the findings of the initial film. Usually this is a request for a T-tube cholangiogram because of visualized bilary calculus or calculi. If so, the same procedure as used for operative cholangiography is to be followed. The major difference is the presence of a tube in the shape of a T now in, or partially in, the common hepatic and bile ducts (Figures 6-3, 6-4).

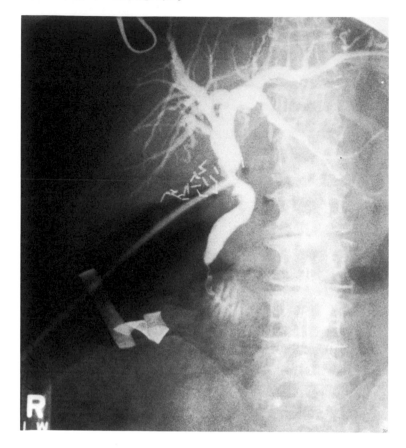

Figure 6-4. An X-ray film of a T-tube cholangiogram.

If the surgeon does not require additional filming after the initial operative cholangiographic study has been returned to the operating room, then the surgical radiologic technologist should take the film to the main X-ray department for immediate viewing by the radiologist. The radiologist will usually give a primary interpretation to be relayed to the surgeon while the operative procedure is still underway.

Operative cholangiography is dependent on efficient cooperation among surgeon, anesthesiologist, and radiologic technologist. It behooves the diligent surgical radiologic technologist to eliminate any confusion by asking pertinent questions and knowing or recognizing all signals or commands prior to making the radiographic exposures. Remember, the patient cannot talk or follow instructions; *he or she is asleep!!!* It is the responsibility of the surgical radiologic technologist to ensure optimum radiographic quality.

SUMMARY

Surgical or operative cholangiography was first performed by Mirizzi in 1930. Operative cholangiography has gained widespread attention and varying degrees of popularity since its inception. Operative cholangiography is based on a combination of surgical and radiologic procedures that will permit radiographic visualization of the biliary tract.

The bile ducts are divided into three major portions: the cystic, the common hepatic, and the common bile, including its terminal portion at the ampulla of Vater. The minor portions include the right and left hepatic ducts with their corresponding radicles.

The operative patient should be positioned for the radiographic examination prior to being anesthetized. A cassette tunnel is employed for use when centering the grid cassette under the patient. The biliary tract is visualized during operative cholangiography by injection of contrast media through a catheter placed in the cystic duct. Suspension of the patient's respiration is required for optimum image results.

Communication for instructions must take place with the surgeon or anesthesiologist prior to radiographic exposure. The surgical radiologic technologist must eliminate the possibility of confusion by knowing all verbal and signal commands.

The initial operative film should be submitted to the surgeon prior to taking the film to the main X-ray department, as additional filming may be required. Additional filming, if required, usually takes the form of an operative T-tube cholangiogram. T-tube cholangiography differs from operative cholangiography in that T-tube cholangiography requires the presence of a rubber tube in the form of a "T" placed through the cystic duct remnant into the common hepatic and bile ducts. The radiographic procedure of T-tube cholangiography does not differ from that of operative cholangiography.

QUESTIONS

1. Surgical or operative cholangiography was first performed by _____ .

2. How long has operative cholangiography been performed?

3. On what is operative cholangiography based?

4. Name the three major portions of the bile ducts.
   1. _____
   2. _____
   3. _____

5. By what method is the biliary tract visualized during operative cholangiography?

6. How is the grid cassette placed under the patient during the surgical procedure?

7. Why should the initial radiograph of an operative cholangiogram be submitted to the surgeon and not the radiologist?

8. How does operative T-tube cholangiography differ from operative cholangiography?

9. Who has the **ultimate** responsibility to ensure that apnea has been induced when performing operative cholangiography?

10. How many degrees of obliquity should be used when positioning the patient for operative cholangiography?

7

Urinary Tract Surgical Radiography

Urinary tract radiography is the most common surgical **Notes** radiographic procedure performed by the surgical radiologic technologist. Unequivocally, the surgical radiologic technologist will perform more urinary radiography than all other surgical radiography combined, exclusive of surgical orthopaedics. Therefore, it is fitting that this chapter consider in some detail the proper procedure in performing the many surgical radiographic urinary examinations.

Urinary tract surgical radiography is divided into three main groups, with subdivisions of the first group. The three main groups are: (1) retrograde pyelography; (2) cystography; and (3) urethrography.

Before the description of retrograde pyelography is given, a short digression is needed to describe the technique of intravenous pyelography (IVP).[1]

Though intravenous pyelography is performed for various purposes and in various manners, it is in simple terms, a diagnostic procedure in which a water-soluble contrast material is injected into a vein to outline the upper urinary tract and the bladder. Then, of course, a series of X-ray films are taken. There are instances when particular patients cannot tolerate

[1]Intravenous pyelography is synonymous with the term intravenous urography.

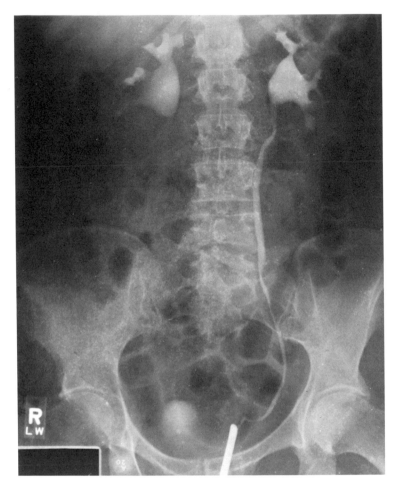

Figure 7-1. Radiograph demonstrating the outline of the calices, renal pelvis, and ureter.

an IVP because of contrast reactions or other reasons. Whatever the reason, the surgeon may decide that the urinary tract must be visualized and decide to perform a radiographic urinary tract examination by the retrograde method. The examination is then referred to as a retrograde pyelogram, a diagnostic procedure in which the surgeon, usually a urologist, passes an optical instrument into the bladder to guide a fine hollow tube, a catheter, into the ureter up to one or both

kidneys. He then injects contrast material to outline the calices, **Notes**
renal pelvis, and ureter and obtains radiographs subsequently
to demonstrate these structures (Figure 7-1).

Strictly speaking, the term pyelogram in itself means only
the delineation of the renal pelvis. However, so as not to
confuse the beginning student, the term pyelogram will be
used in its most common meaning, that is, radiographic
demonstration of the calices, renal pelvis, and ureters.

Like operative cholangiography, surgical urinary tract radiography is a procedure requiring communication and cooperation between the surgeon and the surgical radiologic
technologist. There are many clues unknowingly and know-
ingly given by the urologist and the surgical team that will
enable the surgical radiologic technologist to anticipate action
required of the technologist. These clues are in the form of
verbal orders to the scrub nurse by the surgeon during the
procedure, a particular instrument readied for use by the
surgeon, and/or certain definite movements by the surgeon or
surgical team, to name a few.

Whenever the surgical radiologic technologist can correctly
anticipate the surgeon's needs during a surgical-radiologic
procedure, the surgical radiologic technologist becomes an
asset to the surgical team. After the surgical radiologic
technologist has worked with and assisted the surgeon several
times these clues will become quite apparent. Many urologists
will fill the syringe with contrast media at the outset of the
examination; others will fill the syringe only preparatory to
injection. Some urologists will place the catheter nipple on the
cystoscope just prior to injection whereas others will localize
the cystoscope prior to bladder placement. As stated previously, there are many clues to aid the technologist so that he
or she will know when to prepare for an exposure. Some are
quite apparent and some are learned through experience by
repeatedly working with the same urologist or surgeon. The
surgical radiologic technologist should learn to identify these
clues and strive to become an integral member of the surgical
team.

The surgical team increases in numbers when the urologic
patient is to be surgically examined while under an anesthetic
agent. Most surgical teams consist of a urologist, scrub nurse,
and anesthesiologist, and a surgical radiologic technologist
when performing retrograde pyelography or cystography

Occasionally a second scrub nurse will be in attendance. Many of the cysto rooms are small and crowded with equipment, and, given the presence of a full surgical team, the surgical radiologic technologist must often view the proceedings from the X-ray control booth or some other vantage point. Usually from these positions all conversation can be easily heard and all meaningful actions observed, yet one less person is present to add to an already overcrowded room. There are, of course, many surgical suites that afford large, well-planned cysto rooms that will accommodate everyone on the surgical team, and in such cases rather close observation of the procedure is permitted, if not encouraged.

The previously mentioned urologic examinations, that is, retrograde pyelography, cystography, and urethrography are all performed in what is termed the Cysto Room. The procedure termed cystography is also referred to as "observation cystoscopy" but with a radiographic study. Therefore, radiographic visualization of the urinary bladder by means of contrast medium is termed cystography (Figure 7-2).

The examination is a simple procedure. Cystograms can be obtained by filling the bladder with contrast medium through a urethral catheter and performing subsequent filming. This examination calls for "plain" or "scout" film to be taken prior to introduction of catheter or contrast medium. The size cassette used for the scout film is somewhat determined by the information being sought. Often the surgeon will be interested in ureteral reflux, which precludes the use of a small film that will demonstrate only the urinary bladder and immediate area. A 14 × 17 size film should be used when the demonstration of reflux is desired. Film of this size will be sufficient to demonstrate the entire urinary tract, and if reflux of contrast into the ureters is present there is little possibility of not demonstrating the renal pelvis (Figure 7-3).

The position of the patient and films for cystography is as follows:

The patient is placed in the supine position with the arms and hands at the patient's side. Center the medial sagittal plane of the body to the midline of the table. It is most important that the student radiologic technologist not confuse the centering of the film for scout film of the abdomen for cystography with that of a standard abdominal examination (Figure 7-4).

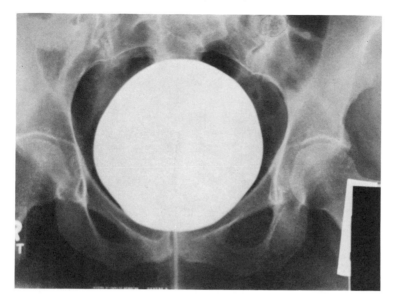

Figure 7-2. An X-ray film of a cystogram.

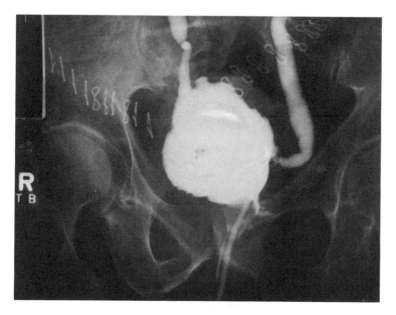

Figure 7-3. An X-ray film of a cystogram demonstrating reflux.

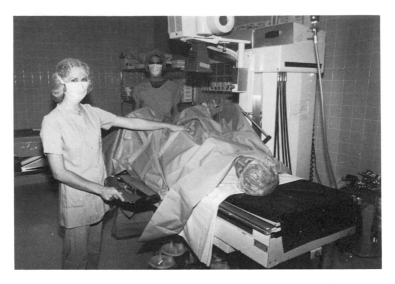

Figure 7-4. Scout film of the abdomen for cystography. Note technologist finger placed on pubic symphysis so that base of cassette can be positioned below this point, It is the expressed opinion of the author that the method of centering the cassette for KUB (kidney, ureter, and bladder) or abdominal radiography as currently taught is inadequate and antiquated.

Place the base of the film 1.5 inches below the pubic symphysis. The central ray is then directed perpendicular to the midpoint of the film. Often the surgeon will require both obliques and a lateral projection of the bladder during the definitive filming. In addition to the oblique and lateral films, the surgeon will often request a postvoiding film with or without obliques.

It is of value to explain the difference of cassette positioning for a KUB (kidney, ureter, and bladder) for the abdomen as opposed to a KUB for cystography. It has been, and currently is, taught that the cassette or film should be centered at the level of the iliac crest. This is often inadequate as a result of differences in anatomy of different patients. This method and position sometimes result in the urinary bladder not being completely demonstrated on the film. The anatomy of many patients is such that the lower portion of the urinary bladder lies inferior to the public symphysis, and often the entire bladder is not demonstrated when the cassette is centered at the iliac crest. The urinary bladder is, however, always demonstrated when the base of the film is placed below the pubic symphysis, as described above. Therefore, it is not only logical to position the film in this manner when performing cystography, but it is correct.

The last division of surgical urography is that of urethrography. Urethrography is, by definition, the radiographic visualization of the urethra with opaque contrast medium. The method of introduction of contrast medium and subsequent filming of the urethra is a relatively easy task if film preparations are carried out before filming.

Contrast medium is introduced into the urinary bladder by means of a catheter. The bladder is allowed to be filled until the patient expresses discomfort. When the bladder is full, the surgeon removes the catheter and the patient is instructed to urinate. The surgical radiologic technologist makes an X-ray exposure when a "full stream" of urine is seen. The patient is placed in the RPO or LPO position with a towel present to absorb the urine, and an exposure is made. The patient is instructed to discontinue urination and then is placed in the lateral position and the procedure is repeated.

More often that not, urethrography is performed as a joint study. That is, urethrography and cystography are performed simultaneously. When performed in this manner, the examination is referred to as a "cystourethrogram" or a "voiding cystourethrogram."

Cystourethrography, or voiding cystourethrography, entails the introduction of a catheter into the urinary bladder and the infusion of radiopaque contrast medium through the catheter, as does urethrography. However, in this procedure, films are obtained of the contrast-filled bladder, as well as the films of the urethra during voiding described above. Because of the presence of the catheter, the examination is properly referred to as a retrograde cystourethrogram. More commonly, however, the examination is simply referred to as a "cystourethrogram," or a "voiding cystourethrogram," as previously stated (Figure 7-5). The student should be aware that urethrography is not necessarily performed as an adjunct to cystography. In fact, one study complements the other, and the student should be well schooled on the technical aspects of both examinations.

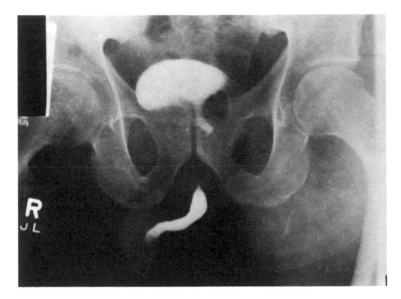

Figure 7-5. Voiding cystourethrography demonstrating the male urethra in a trauma patient.

SUMMARY

Urinary tract radiography is truly the most common surgical radiographic procedure performed by the surgical radiologic technologist.

Urinary tract radiography is divided into three main groups: retrograde pyelography, cystography, and urethrography. Intravenous pyelography is a diagnostic procedure in which a contrast material is injected into a vein to outline the upper urinary tract and the bladder.

Retrograde pyelography is achieved by the passage of a catheter into the ureter(s) and subsequent radiographic filming after the introduction of contrast medium.

Radiographic visualization of the urinary bladder by means of contrast medium is termed cystography.

Urethrography is, by definition, the radiographic visualization of the urethra with opaque contrast medium.

QUESTIONS

1. What is the difference between intravenous pyelography and retrograde pyelography?

2. What is the term used to describe the radiographic demonstration of the calices, renal pelvis, and ureters?

3. What is the term synonymous with cystography?

4. What is the definition of urethrography?

5. What is the term used to describe a joint study of cystography and urethrography?

6. What is the difference between cystography and urethrography?

7. What are the three main groups of urinary tract radiography?

8. What are the reasons that using the iliac crests as a centering reference can be faulty when performing urographic studies?

9. By what means is contrast medium introduced into the bladder during intravenous pyelography?

8

Equipment Safety in the Operating Room

The surgical radiologic technologist has in recent years been called upon to become more involved than in previous years in patient protection, as it concerns the X-ray apparatus in the surgical arena.

In analyzing patient protection from faulty X-ray equipment two distinct yet closely allied hazards must be studied. The first is that of electrical shock. The second is that of explosion.

Electrical shock can occur anywhere; it is not restricted to the operating room. In the operating room, however, a different and potentially more dangerous situation is in effect. Let us consider for a moment the surgical patient undergoing an operation of the slightest magnitude. It is a fact that a human body is "catapulted" through the air when a HIGH VOLTAGE-LOW AMPERAGE shock is sustained. The opposite occurs when a LOW VOLTAGE-HIGH AMPERAGE shock is sustained: the body remains stationary (decidedly so). Therefore, the potentially devastating effects of a patient being electrically shocked by a faulty X-ray machine while undergoing an operation are evident.

Sterile instruments surround the operating room table and hence the patient and may be scattered about the room. The surgical team performing the operation is by necessity in physical contact with the patient, so that the possibility of an electrical shock chain reaction exists, with the potential for killing the entire surgical team.

The second hazard initially is also present in the form of electricity. However, the ramifications can be far more devastating. In the practice of modern anesthesia, explosive anesthetic agents are often used. They include cyclopropane and ether. When either agent is used a potential for explosion exists. When cyclopropane or ether reaches a certain concentration, an explosion set off by a "spark" may occur. Therefore, the surgical radiologic technologist must be constantly on guard for insulation breaks or defects in the external wiring of the X-ray machine. A daily inspection of the insulation should be rigorously carried out so as to preclude the potential for electrical shock or explosion.

SUMMARY

In analyzing patient protection from faulty X-ray machines, two distinct hazards must be considered.

Electrical shock and explosion of volatile anesthetic agents are constant potential operating room hazards, and both may be brought about by faulty wiring insulation on the X-ray apparatus. Either may be fatal to the patient, the members of the surgical team, and even the surgical radiologic technologist. The technologist, therefore, has good reason to maintain the electrical safety of the equipment he uses.

QUESTIONS

1. Describe the effect of high voltage-low amperage shock.

2. Describe the effect of low voltage-high amperage shock.

3. What are the two potentially explosive anesthetic agents?

4. What is the catalyst for such explosions?

9

Hip Nailing Radiography

The use of hip nailing radiography in the operating suite is probably second in frequency only to operative cholangiography and retrograde pyelography. While it is second in frequency to these exams, it is by no means any less important.

Several methods of hip nailing radiography are in use today. The most widely utilized is the "two-tube method." The "two-tube method" involves the use of two portable X-ray machines, or two overhead mounts, that are positioned at right angles to each other (Figure 9-1). It must be remembered that, in order to maintain aseptic technique, all cables must be kept at a safe distance, so as not to come into contact with the patient or his/her sterile drapes.

The patient is placed on a fracture table (such as an Albee) and, after anesthesia has been administered, the surgeon reduces the hip fracture. Time is an important factor in this procedure. Usually the patient with a fractured hip is older, often with some impairment of the heart and/or respiratory system. Such a patient often cannot tolerate a long period of general anesthesia. Therefore, the least amount of time utilized without sacrificing good technique is an important goal in this procedure. The technologist should have the X-ray apparatus ready for immediate positioning as soon as reduction has been completed.

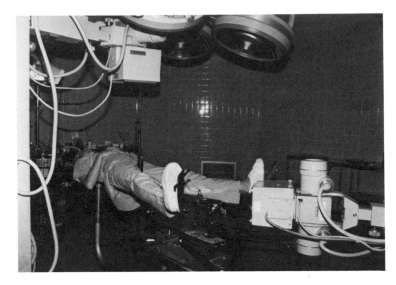

Figure 9-1. Two portable X-ray machines positioned for hip nailing radiography.

The patient is placed in the supine position and the anterior-posterior projection is radiographed exactly as the anterior-posterior projection is in the X-ray department; that is, with the central ray passing through the highest point of the greater trochanter, as shown in Figure 9-2.

The lateral projection is radiographed somewhat differently from the lateral hip X-ray in the X-ray department or even from the portable hip examination on the ward. Fortunately, the surgeon has done most of the hard work of positioning just by reducing the fractured hip. With the legs spread at wide angles to each other, it becomes very easy to move the X-ray tube in between them and, without any patient complaints (because of anesthesia), the tube head may rest against the unaffected hip. Care must be taken to place a towel or sponge between the tube head and the patient's skin so that a thermal burn does not occur. This method is much like a Danelius-Miller modification of Lorenz position except that the unaffected leg does not rest on top of the X-ray tube. Since the unaffected leg is straight and tractioned out, that is, abducted, it cannot be bent to rest on the X-ray tube, since the construction of the Albee table is such that the patient is in a relatively comfortable

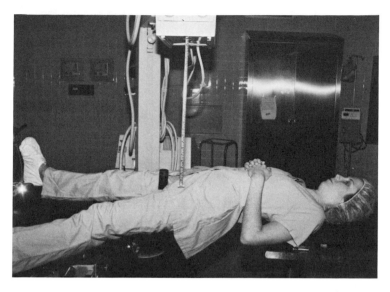

Figure 9-2. Anterior-posterior projection of the right hip for hip nailing radiography with the portable X-ray machine.

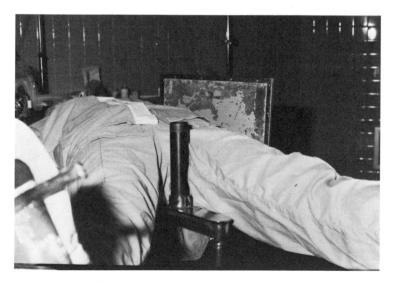

Figure 9-3. Lateral hip projection for hip nailing radiography. Note vertical position of cassette.

Notes

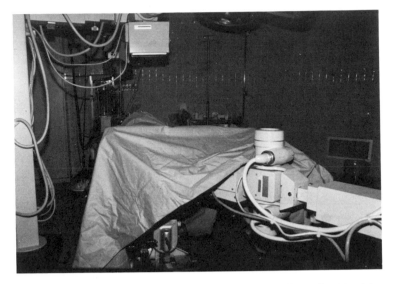

Figure 9-4. Anterior-posterior and lateral position of patient for hip nailing radiography with portable X-ray machines in place.

position. The cassette should be placed in the vertical position and locked in a cassette stand holder as shown in Figure 9-3.

In our department, X-ray cassettes with an 8 to 1 ratio and fast speed screens are used for this examination.

When using the "two-tube method," it is important to know that the radiographic exposures can vary widely, in large part because of the method of simultaneous exposures utilized by many surgical radiologic technologists. The simultaneous exposure method is best utilized with cross-hatched grid cassettes, but may be utilized with regular 8 to 1 grid cassettes. With any cassettes other than cross-hatched grids, a sub-optimal study will probably result.

Since many hospitals or radiology departments do not have cross-hatched grid cassettes, when performing hip nailing radiography the student will want to familiarize herself/himself with the characteristics of regular grid cassettes. This is particularly important when using the simultaneous exposure method.

The patient is set up and draped in the usual sterile manner (Figure 9-4). The X-ray machines are positioned in such a

manner that the surgical radiologic technologist can reach
both machines at the same time. Once this is accomplished,
the surgical radiologic technologist needs only to position the
AP and lateral cassettes, and then make both exposures
simultaneously. One limitation of this method is that there is
always a certain degree of undesirable scatter radiation, and,
because of this, a less than optimal film will result.

As mentioned earlier in this chapter, the "two-tube method"
of hip nailing radiography is probably the most widely used
procedure. Recently, however, there has been a great insurg-
ence of hip nailing fluoroscopy, because of increasing availa-
bility of the portable or fixed C-arm fluoroscopy unit, which has
essentially revolutionalized surgical hip nailing (Figure 9-5).
The orthopaedic surgeon is now able to reduce fractured hips
under fluoroscopy, which makes possible the reduction of the
fracture to such a degree that the postsurgical hip nailing
patient may ambulate weeks earlier than would be allowed
without a fracture that had been reduced to nearly anatomic
perfection.

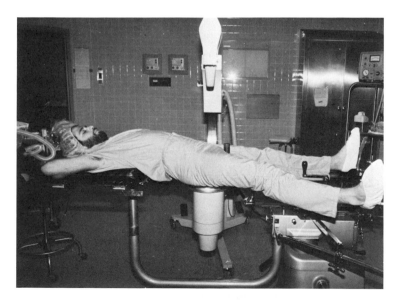

Figure 9-5. The mobile C-arm unit in position for hip nailing
radiography.

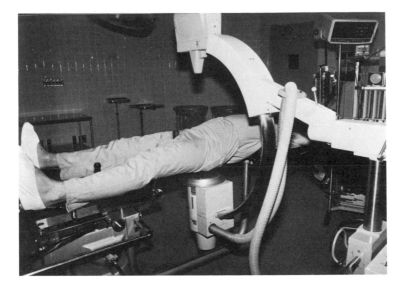

Figure 9-6. C-arm unit used with Albee surgical table.

The position of the C-arm fluoroscopic unit, when perform-ing hip nailing surgery, is varied. There are two very popular methods of positioning the C-arm. The method of positioning of the C-arm depends entirely on the type of operating table used.

The more modern tables are designed to allow the C-arm to be positioned between the patient's legs and, therefore, the bulk of the machine is out of the surgeon's immediate working area (Figure 9-6). The "C" is rotated back and forth to obtain an anterior-posterior and a lateral hip position.

The second method is not so widely used as the first but works as well and, in many cases, perhaps affords a better aseptic technique. It is used with the older fracture tables, such as the Albee table. Many hospitals cannot afford the added expense of a modern table, which can cost up to $20,000, and therefore elect to use the older table which most already possess. This method has the C-arm fluoroscopic unit posi-tioned on the same side of the patient as the hip being repaired. The C-arm fluoroscopic unit from necessity is placed to the left of the surgeon when performing a right hip nailing procedure and to the right of the surgeon when performing a

left hip nailing procedure. The machine is positioned just **Notes**
slightly behind the surgeon (Figure 9-7) The C-arm fluoroscopic unit is separated from the surgeon as well as from the
patient's wound by means of a large drape sheet hung over a
bar running obliquely in position across the patient (Figure 9-
8). The "C" is then rotated in and out to obtain an anterior-
posterior and lateral hip position as needed (Figure 9-9).

The older tables such as the Albee need but few adjustments
to readily adapt to modern C-arm fluoroscopic use. The seat of
the table is brought as far cephalad as possible, and this
suffices for proper patient and C-arm positioning.

The aseptic technique is superb because the C-arm and the
surgeon are separated by an antibacterial barrier—the large
drape sheet described earlier. The more modern tables can
also utilize this antibacterial barrier of a drape sheet used to
separate the C-arm from the patient, patient's wound, and
surgeon.

Whichever method is used, optimal fluoroscopy and the
integrity of aseptic technique can be achieved.

The modern C-arm fluoroscope coupled with a modern
video recorder offers virtually unlimited radiographic and

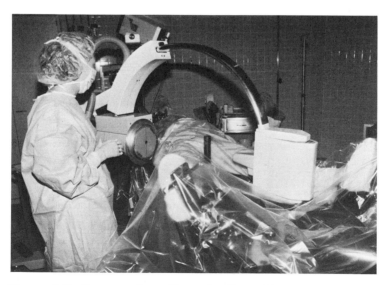

Figure 9-7. C-arm unit positioned adjacent to surgeon.

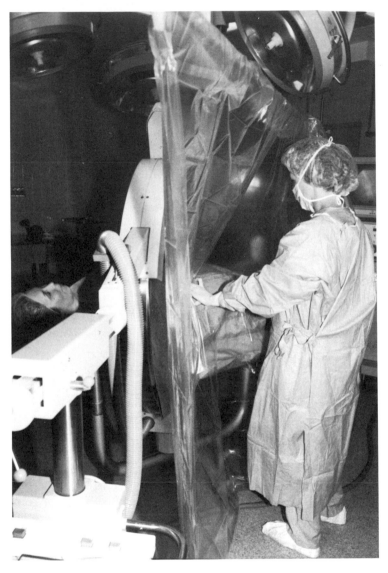

Figure 9-8. C-arm positioned adjacent to surgeon with oblique cross bar affording continuity of sterile integrity.

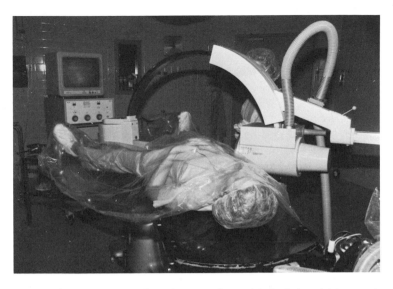

Figure 9-9. The tube head rotated to obtain lateral hip position.

fluoroscopic capabilities to the orthopaedic surgeon. The video recorder in itself is a major time-saver when used in hip nailing procedures. As discussed earlier in Chapter 5, the video recorder has certain features and capabilities that are attractive not only to the surgical radiologic technologist but also to the surgeon. One of these features is the capability to "play-back" the video and have instant visualization of the "scout" frame or earlier frames demonstrating the progress of the hip nailing surgery. In addition, the recorded video images can be transferred to permanent film merely by pressing a button.

The "two-tube method" of hip nailing radiography is the most widely used because most hospitals in this country are small and many cannot afford the luxury of a C-arm fluoroscope. The larger medical centers are usually government subsidized and most possess at least one C-arm fluoroscopic unit, and in many cases, two or more units. It is apparent that even now the smaller hospitals are purchasing the C-arm fluoroscopy unit and it is thought that soon the "two-tube method" of hip nailing radiography will be used only as a "back-up" to the C-arm fluroscopic method.

Although the C-arm unit is capable of producing radiographic exposures, it is generally used only for fluoroscopy. However, many surgeons request radiographic exposures at the beginning, during, or after an operation. The C-arm unit is limited to radiographic exposures of smaller size films. This, of course, is due to the limited arrangement of the physical "C" itself. The usual film size does not exceed 8 inches by 10 inches for exposure by the C-arm.

Surgeons should probably be discouraged in using the C-arm as a radiographic unit. The C-arm unit is designed for fluoroscopic use and to use it routinely for fluoroscopic-radiographic procedures is not optimal utilization of this equipment. Radiographic films for hip nailing procedures should routinely be carried out postoperatively in the recovery room or in the main X-ray department. If done in the recovery room, the standard portable X-ray machine can be used to obtain a permanent record of the procedure. The patient can also be radiographed in the X-ray department on his or her return trip to the ward following release from the recovery room.

SUMMARY

Hip nailing radiography is second in frequency only to operative cholangiography and retrograde pyelography. There are several methods of hip nailing radiography in use today. The "two-tube method" and the C-arm fluroscopic method are both currently used.

The C-arm fluoroscopic unit has essentially revolutionalized modern surgical hip nailing radiography. Orthopaedic surgeons are now reducing fractured hips under fluoroscopy, thereby affording the patient an added service. The C-arm fluroscope coupled with a modern video recorder offers virtually unlimited radiographic and fluoroscopic capabilities to the orthopaedic surgeon. The video recorder in itself is a major time-saver when used in hip nailing procedures. One of the features of the video recorder is the capability to "playback" the video and have instant visualization of the "scout" frame or earlier frames demonstrating the progress of the hip nailing surgery.

The "two-tube method" of hip nailing radiography is the most widely used because most hospitals in the United States are small and many cannot afford the luxury of a C-arm fluoroscope.

Although the C-arm unit is capable of producing radiographic exposures, it is generally used only for fluoroscopy. The C-arm unit is limited to radiographic exposures of smaller size films. This, of course, is because of the limited range of the physical "C" itself. The usual film size does not exceed 8×10 inches for exposure by the C-arm.

QUESTIONS

1. The use of hip nailing radiography in an operating suite is probably second only to _____ .

2. What is the most widely used method of hip nailing radiography?

3. Through what structure does the central ray pass when radiographing the hip in the anterior-posterior position?

4. What method of hip nailing radiography, when using the C-arm, probably affords a better aseptic technique?

5. When using the C-arm fluoroscopic unit with an older fracture table, on what side of the surgeon would the C-arm fluoroscopic unit be placed if the surgeon was performing surgery on the right hip?

6. When using the C-arm fluoroscopic unit with an older fracture table, on what side of the surgeon would the C-arm fluoroscopic unit be placed if the surgeon was performing surgery on the left hip?

7. When using the "two-tube method" for hip nailing radiography and making simultaneous exposures, what type grids are most desirable?

8. Why is the "two-tube method" of hip nailing radiography probably the most widely used method in the United States today?

9. When using the C-arm for surgical hip nailing radiography, it is desirable to separate the machine from the surgeon and by what means?

10. What is the main use of the C-arm: fluoroscopic use or radiographic use?

10

Radiography of Surgical Laminectomies

Because the practice of radiography of surgical laminectomies **Notes**
is on the increase it is appropriate to touch briefly on this
subject. The surgical procedure known as laminectomy has
been performed for some time. Radiography of the surgical
procedure has become relatively common only in the past
several years.

Radiography of surgical laminectomy, whether it be cervical
or lumbar, simply involves radiography of the cervical or
lumbar spine in the true lateral position.

The patient is placed in the prone position on the operating
table when performing lumbar laminectomy (Figure 10-1). The
surgeon requests X-rays of the lumbar spine so that the
placement of a needle in the disc space can be visualized to
determine the correct level and/or area being operated (Figure
10-2). The spine is radiographed in the cross-table lateral
projection. The surgeon will usually show or tell the surgical
radiologic technologist where the needle is placed; it is at this
point demonstrated by the surgeon that the cassette should be
centered. The central ray is then centered to the cassette as
shown in Figure 10-3. Since this study requires the use of a
grid cassette, it must be remembered that central ray centering
is critical. As with all grids the surgical radiologic technologist
must be precise in centering; otherwise grid cutoff will result.

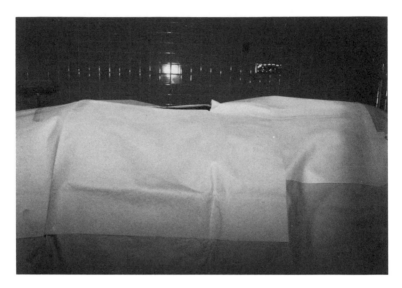

Figure 10-1. Patient in prone position for lumbar laminectomy. Note spinal needle projecting from patient's lumbar area.

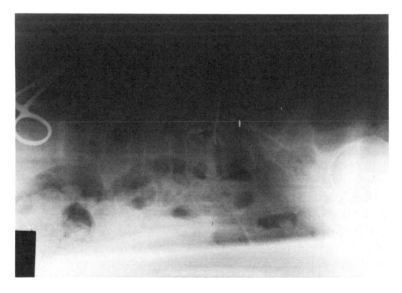

Figure 10-2. An X-ray film demonstrating the probe positioned in interdisc space.

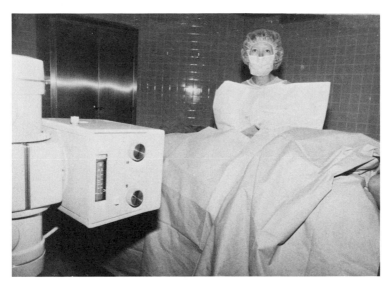

Figure 10-3. Central ray centered to cassette for lateral projection for lumbar laminectomy.

The cervical laminectomy procedure is somewhat different from that of the lumbar in that the patient is usually in the sitting erect position. The patient is placed on the operating table and the table is adjusted in such a manner that the patient merely sits erect.

As with the lumbar laminectomy the surgeon will place a needle in the cervical disc space at the area of interest. The center of the grid cassette is placed at the level of the needle and the central ray directed to the center of the cassette (Figure 10-5).

One of the main difficulties in performing optimum radiography of lumbar or cervical laminectomies lies in the use of the sterile bag that contains the grid cassette and thereby maintains a sterile field. There are many transparent bags that are used to hold cassettes when performing certain types of surgical radiography. With the transparent bags there is little problem in beam alignment, since the cassette can be easily seen (Figure 10-6). However, other bags that are quite popular and used extensively are not transparent and afford only an outline of the cassette (Figure 10-7). The nontransparent type

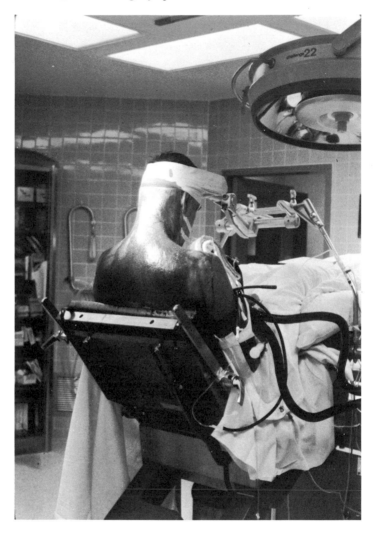

Figure 10-4. Patient in erect sitting position for cervical laminectomy.

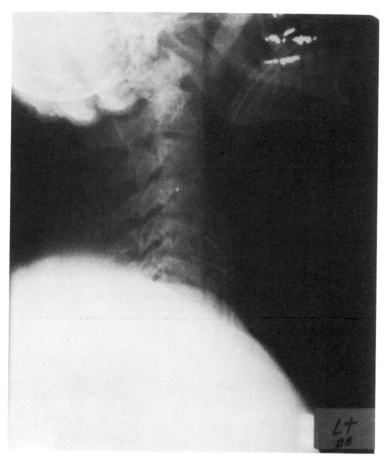

Figure 10-5. X-ray film of cervical laminectomy demonstrating surgical instrument.

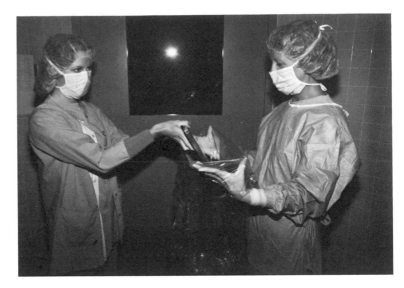

Figure 10-6. Cassette placed in transparent sterile bag.

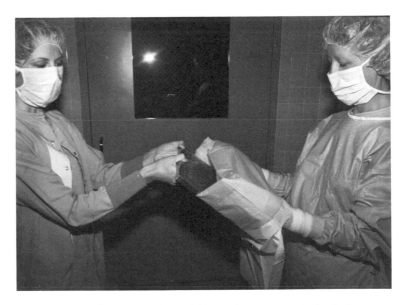

Figure 10-7. Cassette placed in nontransparent sterile bag.

bag is quite sturdy, and, like the transparent bag, will accommodate cassettes of all sizes, including 14×17. Since only an outline of the cassette is afforded with the nontransparent bag, it is important that the beam alignment be accomplished with great care so as not produce grid cutoff. **Notes**

SUMMARY

Radiography of surgical laminectomies, whether cervical or lumbar, has as its goal radiography of the cervical or lumbar spine in the true lateral position. Radiography of surgical laminectomies has become prevalent only during the last 2 or 3 years.

The lumbar spine is radiographed at the area of needle insertion for lumbar laminectomies and the cervical spine is radiographed in the lateral position at the area of the needle insertion to demonstrate the exact placement in the intervertebral disc. The lumbar spine is radiographed with the patient in the prone position and with a cross-table lateral spine projection.

The surgeon will usually show or tell the surgical radiologic technologist the area of needle placement. Because of the use of grid cassettes, care must be taken with central beam alignment so as to prohibit grid cutoff.

One of the main difficulties of performing radiography of surgical laminectomies is the use of nontransparent bags that are used as cassette holders.

QUESTIONS

1. What is the purpose of radiographing surgical laminectomies?

2. What position is the patient in on the operating table for a lumbar laminectomy?

3. What radiographic view is obtained for lumbar laminectomies?

4. What position is the patient in on the operating table for a cervical laminectomy and what radiographic view is obtained for cervical laminectomies?

5. What is the main problem for the surgical radiologic technologist in obtaining optimum radiographs for lumbar or cervical laminectomyies?

11

Radiography of Surgical Lithotomy

The word *lith* is a Greek word meaning *stone*. Lithotomy is the removal of a stone or calculus from a duct or organ. Although the surgical radiologic technologist is not frequently called on to participate in surgical lithotomy, when required, he or she usually plays an important role in the lithotomy procedure.

Surgical lithotomy usually involves removal of: (1) bladder calculi; (2) ureteral calculi, (3) calculi in the renal pelvis or calyces. The surgical radiologic technologist is seldom called on to radiograph lithotomy of the bladder. However, when his or her services are needed in this situation, it is to perform a bladder radiography and this is performed in the same manner as a routine KUB with the exception of the film size. The patient is placed in the anterior posterior supine position on the operating table as shown in Figure 11-1. A 10×12 cassette is used and is positioned with the base of the film 1½ inches inferior to the pubic symphysis. The central ray is then directed at the center of the cassette (Figure 11-2).

Ureteral calculi present a much different problem. If the ureter contains a stone in the distal third of the ureter then basket extraction is utilized (Figure 11-3). If the calculus is superior to the distal third of the ureter then ureterolithotomy is performed. Often, even if the calculus is in the distal third of the ureter, basket extraction cannot be achieved.

97

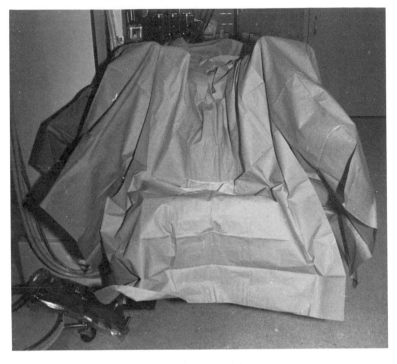

Figure 11-1. Patient in lithotomy position.

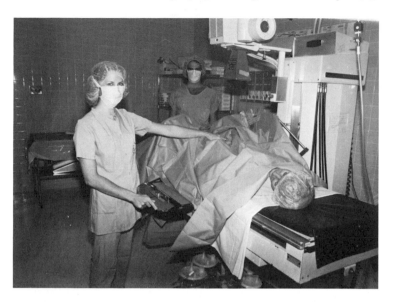

Figure 11-2. Scout film of the abdomen. Note technologist's finger placed on pubic symphysis so that base of cassette can be positioned below this point.

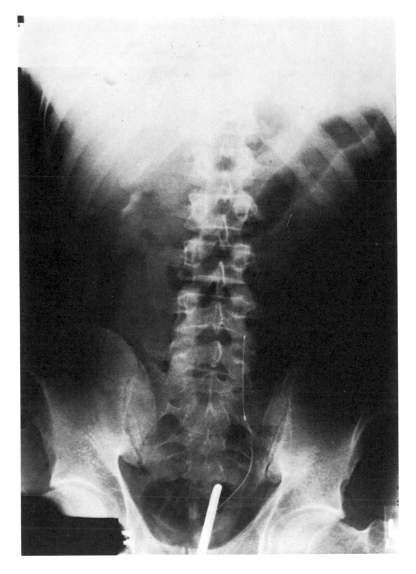

Figure 11-3. KUB with basket extraction catheter in ureter.

Let us consider basket extraction surgery and hence basket extraction radiography. As previously mentioned, if a calculus is located or contained in the distal portion of the distal third of the ureter, the surgeon will usually attempt to remove the ureteral stone by means of a catheter with a built in wire mesh basket. The basket is contained within the catheter and when manipulated by the surgeon the basket is pushed through the catheter and opens inside the ureter (Figures 11-4A and B). This then allows the surgeon to try to capture the calculus with the basket, thereby avoiding ureteral surgery. The surgical radiologic technologist is called on to perform what is termed basket extraction radiography. Basket extraction radiography is nothing more than a retrograde urinary study as described in Chapter 7. The patient is placed on a cysto table in the usual manner (i.e., with legs in stirrups) and a KUB is obtained (Figure 11-5). The surgeon may inject a radiopaque contrast material to delineate better the stone contained in the ureter. Many times the surgeon will not use a contrast material but instead may request only a "scout" or plain film of the abdomen, or KUB. In either case, the study performed is that of an abdominal radiography.

If the ureteral calculus is contained superior to the distal third of the ureter then the usual procedure is termed ureterolithotomy. Ureterolithotomy is incision of the ureter and subsequent removal of the calculus. As a rule, the surgical radiologic technologist is not called on to perform any radiographic examination during this procedure.

The third aspect of surgical lithotomy is that of pyelolithotomy. Because of the infrequency of this procedure, the surgical radiologic technologist probably experiences more problems with this than with any other surgical radiographic study performed.

Pyelolithotomy is the removal of a calculus or of calculi from the kidney itself. The patient is placed in the lithotomy position on the operating table (Figure 11-6). The radiographic procedure is difficult at best because of the complete loss of the sight of the film packet. The film used for pyelolithotomy is called KS film (Kodak) and is packaged with two films inside a black plastic container (Figure 11-7). This packet is sterilized prior to the schedule surgery and is brought into the operating

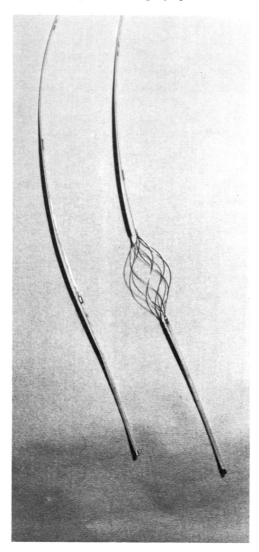

Figure 11–4A

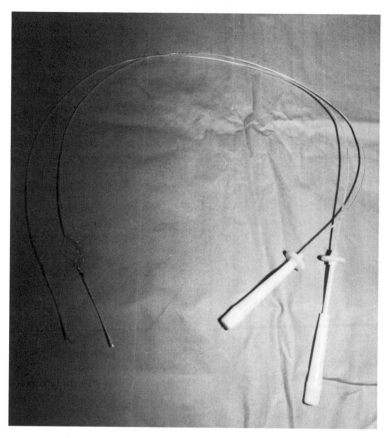

Figure 11-4A and B. Photographs of basket extraction catheter. Note basket extending from tip of catheter.

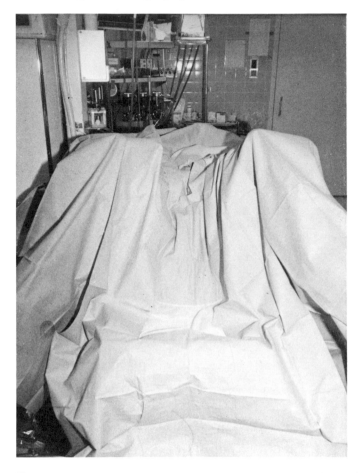

Figure 11-5. Patient in stirrups in preparation for urinary study.

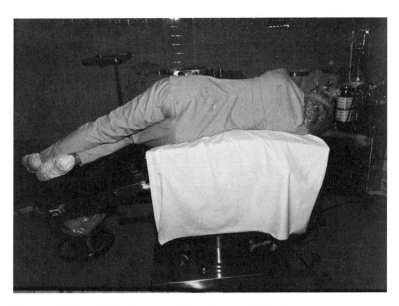

Figure 11-6. Patient in position for pyelolithotomy.

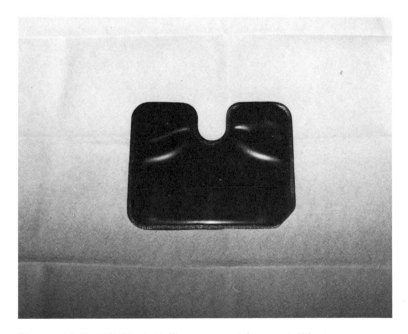

Figure 11-7. KS (Kodak) film as used for pyelolithotomy.

room at the beginning of the surgery. The surgeon places the packet **inside** the patient's body and then covers the sterile wound with a surgical towel. The surgical radiologic technologist then obtains X-ray films of the kidney that has been placed on top of the film packet.

The surgical radiologic technologist should watch carefully and pay close attention to the position of the film packet, as the angle of the X-ray tube depends entirely on the position of the film packet. After radiographic exposure of the film the packet is opened and the film can be processed through the automatic processor by butt splicing the ends to a larger film or by simply processing the KS film as it exists. The resulting radiograph shows the number and position of stones in the kidney.

SUMMARY

The term lithotomy means the removal of a stone of calculus from a duct or organ. Surgical lithotomy is utilized for the removal of (1) bladder calculi; (2) ureteral calculi; and (3) renal calculi.

Basket extraction and hence basket extraction radiography is utilized when a stone is contained in the distal portion of the distal third of the ureter.

KS (Kodak) film is used when performing pyelolithotomy.

QUESTIONS

1. What are the main three types of urinary lithotomy?

2. What radiographic view is taken for a basket extraction procedure?

3. What view is taken for a bladder lithotomy?

4. What type film is used for pyelolithotomy?   **Notes**

5. Where in the ureter must a stone be contained before basket extraction is usually attempted?

12

Surgical Arteriography

The most common surgical arteriogram is that of femoral
arteriography. Many surgeons use a C-arm fluoroscopic unit
with this procedure, but the use of a simple ceiling-mounted
X-ray tube or a portable X-ray machine is more common.

The patient is placed on the operating table in the supine
position and the leg in question is usually supported at the
knee by a sterile basin or towel. (The basin or towel is removed
for the arteriogram study) (Figure 12-1).

The radiographic procedure itself is little more than lateral or
oblique views of the femur. The C-arm, when used, offers the
surgeon a limited viewing area due to the physical limitations
of the fluoroscopic unit. Again, some surgeons use the C-arm
fluoroscope, but the portable X-ray unit is the machine of
choice. When using the C-arm fluoroscopic unit, the unit is
positioned with the image intensifier over the anastomotic site
(Figure 12-2).

The procedure when using the portable X-ray unit differs
greatly from that using the C-arm fluoroscope. A 14 × 17 grid
cassette is placed in a sterile bag container and placed
diagonally under the patient's leg (the diagonal positioning of
the cassette allows the greatest possible length of artery to be
included on the film) (Figure 12-3). The problem of using
nontransparent bags again arises, with the possibility of poor

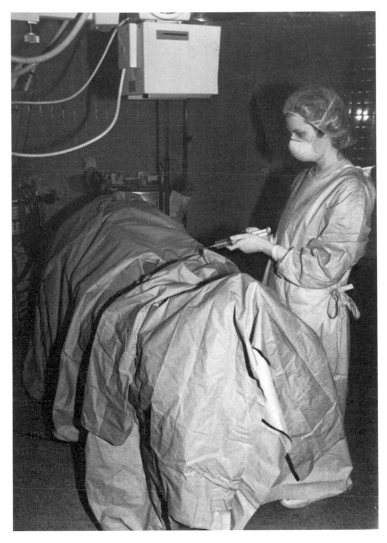

Figure 12-1. Patient in position for surgical femoral arteriography with utilization of a portable X-ray machine.

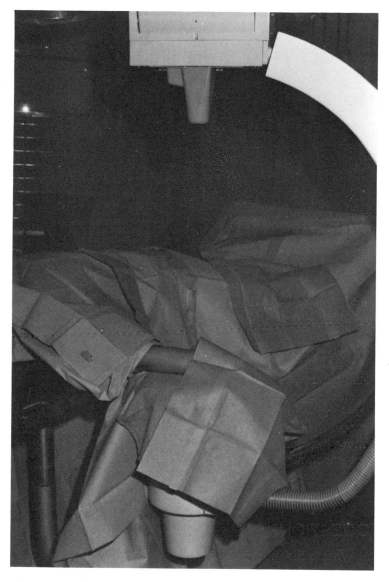

Figure 12-2. Patient in position for surgical arteriography of the arm with utilization of C-arm mobile unit.

Notes

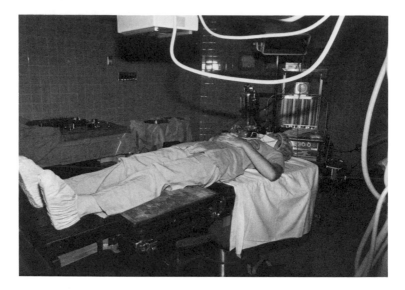

Figure 12-3. Grid cassette placed under patient's leg for surgical femoral arteriography.

beam alignment and consequent grid cutoff. (See Chapter 10, Radiography of Surgical Laminectomies.)

Most surgeons prefer a long radiographic exposure time so that the entire vascular graft can be visualized. A long exposure time allows the demonstration of not only the arterial phase but also the venous phase; a 1½–3 second exposure is not uncommon.

QUESTIONS

1. What is the most common type of surgical radiography?

2. What is the X-ray apparatus of choice when performing surgical arteriography?

3. Why is the C-arm fluoroscopic unit used sparingly in the surgical arteriogram procedure?

4. What are the desired radiographic exposure times for surgical femoral arteriography?

5. What radiographic view is obtained when performing surgical femoral arteriography?

13

Radiography of Surgical Reduction of Fractures of the Extremities

The surgical radiologic technologist, as mentioned before, will perform more orthopaedic surgical radiography than any other single procedure. In fact, orthopaedic surgical radiography may be utilized as much or more than all other surgical radiologic procedures combined.

There are many facets to orthopaedic surgical radiography: hip nailing radiography, surgical laminectomies, zygomatic repairs; the list is practically endless. The greater part of orthopaedic surgical radiography, however, involves radiography of surgical reduction of fractures of the extremities—both open and closed reductions.

The student surgical radiologic technologist needs to have a clear understanding of beam angulation and alignment prior to attempting surgical extremity radiography. This knowledge is important because of the problem of bone elongation owing to central ray angulation. While an anterior posterior view of the elbow or other bony structures may indeed be an anterior posterior view, it may be suboptimal and misleading to the surgeon if there is elongation of the particular part being repaired. The student, as well as the experienced surgical radiologic technologist, will face many situations where a particular view seems **impossible** because of the patient's position; however, in most cases, a very close approximation to the desired view can be obtained with proper manipulation of

Notes

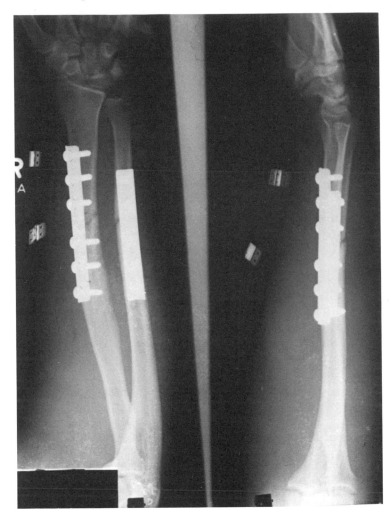

Figure 13-1. An x-ray film of internal European compression plates in a patient's forearm.

the X-ray tube. Again, the importance of obtaining films with the least possible radiographic distortion must be stressed, and this depends directly on proper beam alignment.

Many open reductions of the extremities include metal screw placement. This often appears on the surgery schedule as "internal fixation" or "internal screw fixation." Internal screw fixation simply means the strategic placement of metal screws to repair, reduce, or fix bone in a certain position (Figure 13-1).

Closed reduction extremity radiography is different than open reduction in that the skin is not surgically opened. The extremity is merely repaired by pressure on the extremity, whether it be a pulling or pushing motion. There are occasions when metal screw fixation is performed without opening the skin. In these cases the screw is drilled through the skin into the bone. (Some ankle, wrist, and elbows are repaired in this manner.)

The C-arm fluoroscopic unit is playing a greater role in the surgical reduction of extremities due to the time saving factor. On many occasions the surgeon needs only to have a brief look at the extremity being repaired and this is easily accomplished by the use of the aforementioned C-arm unit.

In conclusion, it must be remembered that most of the open reduction extremity repair work will require the use of a plastic bag to contain the cassette, and, as mentioned throughout this text, the surgical radiologic technologist must be extremely careful if the bag is nontransparent to align the tube correctly.

SUMMARY

The surgical radiologic technologist will perform more orthopaedic surgical radiography than any other single procedure. The greater part of this orthopaedic surgical radiography will involve radiography of surgical repair of fractured extremities—both open and closed reduction.

A clear understanding and knowledge of beam alignment is essential to avoid bone elongation. Many open reductions of the extremities include metal screw placement. Closed reduction extremity radiography is different from open reduction in that the skin is not surgically opened.

Notes

The C-arm flouroscopic unit is playing a greater role in surgical reduction of the extremities because of to the time-saving factor.

QUESTIONS

1. What is the greater part of orthopaedic surgical radiography that the surgical radiologic technologist will be called on to perform?

2. What does the term "open reduction" mean? Explain.

3. What does the term "closed reduction" mean? Explain.

4. How is bone elongation minimized?

5. Why is the C-arm fluoroscopic unit playing a greater role in open and closed reduction of the upper and lower extremities?

Index

119